RXpert SERIES
Student's Companion

Computer-Aided Drug Development

RXpert SERIES
Student's Companion

Computer-Aided Drug Development

Amaresh Prusty
M.Pharm, Ph.D.
Associate Professor,
Royal College of Pharmacy and Health Sciences,
Berhampur, Odisha. 760 002.

PharmaMed Press
An imprint of BSP Books Pvt. Ltd.
4-4-309/316, Giriraj Lane,
Sultan Bazar, Hyderabad - 500 095.

Computer-Aided Drug Development
by **Amaresh Prusty**

Published by:

Pharma Med PRESS An Imprint of BSP Books Pvt. Ltd.

™ **PharmaMed Press**

An imprint of BSP Books Pvt. Ltd.
4-4-309/316, Giriraj Lane, Sultan Bazar, Hyderabad - 500 095.
Phone: 040-23445688; Fax: 91+40-23445611
e-mail: info@pharmamedpress.com
www.pharmamedpress.com/pharmamedpress.net

ISBN: 9978-93-48734-22-8 (Hardback)

Preface

It is an immense pleasure to bring out the First Edition of book titled "Computer-Aided Drug Development," which is dedicated to the faculty and students of both B. Pharma and M. Pharma. Sincere efforts have been made to present theoretical aspects in detail for easy understanding on the pivotal role how computers play in shaping various aspects of drug discovery, formulation, and characterization. The major objective of this book is to provide students with collective information about the subject in simple and lucid language.

The book contains five units, where a comprehensive and detail representation given on fundamental role computers in pharmaceutical research and development, utilization of computational techniques to predict the absorption, distribution, metabolism, and excretion (ADME) profiles of drug candidates along with the role of Artificial Intelligence, Robotics, and Computational Fluid Dynamics in drug development that helps readers to gain insights into the evolution of drug development paradigms and the exciting potential that justify the multifaceted applications of computational techniques in pharmaceutical research exploration.

Author is very much grateful to PharmaMed Press, Hyderabad for all their efforts in publishing this book.

Suggestions and comments are always welcome and they shall be gratefully acknowledged.

- Author

Acknowledgement

I take this opportunity to humbly acknowledge the entire team of Pharma Book Syndicate, An Imprint of BSP Books Pvt. Ltd. for giving me the opportunity to write this book. A few years back, I was involved in writing a chapter of a book for the M. Pharmacy PCI syllabus, but this is the first time I have been the author of a book published by a reputed publisher. I express my heartfelt gratitude and thankfulness to the Director Prof. P N Murthy, Principal Prof S K Panda, and the management's Royal College of Pharmacy and Health Sciences, Berhampur, for providing all necessary facilities and utilization of the library reference book in completing the preparing the book which is as per New PCI syllabus for M Pharm students with detail and vivid presentations of each topic. Next, I would like to express my deep sense of gratitude to Mrs. Sasmita Kmari Padhi, Lecturer College of Nursing, MKCG, Berhampur, Odisha, for motivating me to write a book and revise the contents meticulously. I feel extreme pleasure in expressing my deep sense of gratitude to Mr. Nikunjesh Shah and Mr. Naresh Davergave for their keen interest and valuable suggestions, active cooperation, and constant encouragement for publishing the book. My sincere thanks to all respected teachers, Prof. B K Gupta, Retd. Professor, Department of Pharmacy, Jadavpur University, Prof Amiyakanta Mishra, and beloved students. Suggestions and comments for further improvement of this book will be appreciated and acknowledged.

Last but not least, I am thankful to Lord Jagannath, my beloved parents, my brother, and my son Shriyans, Baivab, and Shivin.

We are equally thankful to all other BSP Books Pvt Ltd. employees who have contributed to in this book's publication.

- Author

Contents

Unit – II

Computational Modelling of Drug Disposition Simulation Modelling

Unit – III

Concept of Optimization, Optimization Parameters

Unit – IV

Computer Aided Biopharmaceutical Characterization

UNIT I

History of Computers in Pharmaceutical Research

No one can picture living without computers when it comes to storing, sending, and managing information in today's fast-paced world.

The pharmaceutical industry's R&D system also includes computers, which play an essential role in drug discovery, laboratory equipment operation, and processing clinical and experimental data.

Computers first entered the pharmaceutical sector in the 1940s, but their primary usage was for accounting and other non-scientific tasks.

The importance of computers in comprehending the relationship between a molecule's chemical structure and its molecular characteristics, including biological activity, evolves in tandem with the pace of discovery and innovation in the development of new chemical entities or compounds. Calculating molecular characteristics has made theoretical and experimental investigations into molecular structures possible.

Mid-19th Century

Publications presenting mathematical relationships between chemical structure and biological activity started appearing in the middle of the nineteenth century. After much work, QSAR (Quantitative Structure Activity Relationships) was introduced, which essentially used chemical descriptors to describe biological activity. These molecular descriptors only provide a numerical number, either computed or experimental, that characterizes the chemical structure of that particular molecule. The creation and application of QSARs were products of computer engineering. Thus, the computer—originally intended for use in the military and accounting—evolved into a tool for scientific advancement.

The role of computers has emerged as a major tool for analysing voluminous and high-dimensional data in pharmaceutical research, helping to overcome previous barriers to medication discovery.

Researchers want to quicken the pace of drug development and lower associated expenses by tapping into the help of computers. According to Bekryl, a market research organisation, the application of AI in pharmaceutical research might save more than US $70 billion in drug development costs by 2028. By relying on chemists to develop, synthesise, and analyse a large number of compounds without first subjecting them to a broad screening process, rational structure-based drug discovery techniques are gaining popularity.

The early 1960s

Drugs were discovered in the early 1960s via a process of trial and error. Here, the chemists or discoverer would peruse patent literature for competing products, draw on their imagination and experience to create therapeutically active compounds, and then test them for bioactivity against other targets that were being studied at the time or as potential targets in disease treatment by forming complexes with protein compounds. But now in the realm of computer science, AI is considered a branch that focuses on problem-solving using symbolic programming. It has the potential to revolutionize various industries, including pharmacy. A considerable amount of research is being conducted to enhance the current AI technology, aiming to make the pharmacy profession more efficient and effective by discovering new drug molecules along with their formulation and optimization parameters

Early adopters of computational drug discovery included industry heavyweights like Abbott, Schering-Plough, Upjohn, and Dow Chemical. While some of these businesses poured money into software and gear, others educated their own scientists to apply computational chemistry. Eli Lilly was one of the first places computational drug development made headway; there, scientists discovered a link between the antibacterial activity of cephalosporin and the computed electronic structure of its beta-lactam ring. Despite these promising beginnings, some businesses gave up on computational drug development because upper management didn't back their efforts. However, Lilly persisted and eventually established itself as a leader in this field. The company's success was due in part to its investment in computational infrastructure and its willingness to train its scientists in this new technology.

Hardware and software limitations hampered computational drug development in its early stages. Computers were slow and had limited memory, and the software was often difficult to use. However, as computers became more powerful and software became more user-friendly, computational drug discovery became more widespread.

One of the challenges of computational drug discovery is the communication gap between medicinal and computational chemists. Computational chemists are more concerned with the theoretical parts of medication design, while medicinal chemists are more concerned with the practical synthesis and testing of novel chemicals. Because of this, tensions and miscommunications may arise between the two communities. By arranging a number of seminars to educate medicinal chemists on computational drug development, Lilly made a constructive move toward solving this problem. Because of this, there was better communication between the two parties, and they worked together more on medication development.

These days, the drug development process would not be complete without computational drug discovery. Beneficial medication candidates may be discovered and enhanced, and their toxicity can be foreseen using this method. The use of computational drug discovery has the potential to significantly increase the success rate of new medication approvals and decrease the time it takes to create drugs.

The early 1970s

Computational chemists could extract new compounds with therapeutic activity as additional compounds were added to the Protein Data Bank (PDB) and the Cambridge Structural Database (CSD) for research in the 1970s.

In the 1980s, advances were furthered by the creation of the IBM personal computer (PC). In 1984, the Apple Macintosh was developed, and computer software for word processing and graphics was discovered. This software greatly assisted medicinal chemists in readily accessing chemical databases.

Chem Draw and similar programs made it easy for chemists to draw two-dimensional chemical diagrams for use in reports, articles, and patents; in the future, these diagrams will be useful for visualizing the three-dimensional structures of compounds using either a ball and stick model or a computer screen.

Between 1975 and 1985

During this period, the computer-aided Drug Design method was used to study the discovery of a new chemical entity. 48 US-based chemical and pharmaceutical firms that used CAD software participated in the research.

The 1990s

The use of supercomputers in the search for novel illness therapy targets began in the 1990s.

Cray Research's CEO daringly met Lilly's CEO and offered the corporation an enticing price for a supercomputer. His strategy was successful in maintaining a competitive edge in the pharmaceutical marketplace, as numerous pharmaceutical companies—including Merck, Bristol-Myers Squibb, Marion Merrell Dow, Johnson & Johnson, and Bayer—bought or rented supercomputers from Cray Research.

Because of the shift in perspective towards computational chemists brought about by the growing importance of computational drug discovery, businesses like Lilly now include computational chemists as co-inventors on patents in which they have a hand.

Statistical Modelling in Pharmaceutical Research and Development

The pharmaceutical business has effectively used statistical principles and methods to address several difficulties. Due to the high stakes involved, many pharmaceutical firms are hesitant to spend extensively on the quality of their large-scale production processes before a drug's commercialization approval. This is because a negative outcome in a clinical trial might result in the complete failure of the product.

A medicine's patent life may expire between sixty and seventy-five percent throughout the twelve to fifteen years it takes to get from ideation to clinical approval. Phases IIA and IIB clinical studies, which determine the dosage and demonstrate the product's idea, may still be unsuccessful after 40-50% of the product's patent life has passed. Also, Phase I (first-in-human) studies, which evaluate the safety, tolerability, and drug blood levels, are anticipated to fail with one out of three medicines.

Consequently, after the successful completion of Phase III clinical trials, pharmaceutical firms are under significant economic pressure to expedite filing new drug applications (NDAs) with regulatory authorities. When launching a product, a substantial quantity of capital is required. Consequently, substantial "at-risk" development operations may incur losses that might outweigh the time and resources allocated to quality and process knowledge projects.

Although the foundations of statistical theory may be found in developments in probability made in the 18th century, the discipline as we know it today did not form until the latter half of the nineteenth and the beginning of the twentieth century. Charles S. Peirce created a theory of statistical inference in his two books "Illustrations of the Logic of Science" (1877–1878) and "A Theory of Probable Inference" (1883), which highlighted the significance of reasoning based on randomization in statistics. Because the calculations required to do the analysis of variance were so laborious and time-consuming, Fisher started to pay close attention to them in his research on the topic. The Major obstacle that nowadays the pharmaceutical industry is facing is not only developing a new chemical entity but also making it available in the market in a suitable dosage form, as from formulating to marketing requires more time and money. So to solve this problem, pharmaceutical industries are using various in silico modeling or pharmacophore modeling, which helps the industry achieve its objective quickly.

Statistical analysis aims to find trends and patterns in large datasets by gathering, analyzing, and presenting the results. People in research, business, and government use statistics to make better, more informed choices daily. In their day-to-day operations, pharmaceutical companies employ roles ranging from the design of tests to the analysis of drug trials and the sale of medicines. Statistical methods applied to the aforementioned pursuits constitute pharmaceutical statistics.

Stastical Modelling

Breiman gave the concept of stastical modelling, proposing his view that the concept has two parts/cultures: the first part is data modeling, and the other part is algorithmic modeling. It is crucial to use modeling principles in order to comprehend the mechanism, which entails taking a vector of response variables y and a set of input variables x and studying their connection using modeling approaches. The data-generating system under study may be simplified using a model.

Types

Descriptive Modelling

Models like these work great for ruling out competing theories, but they don't do anything at all to understand the phenomenon at work, or the mechanism that generates the data; all they do is offer a reasonable description of the data in the right format.

Mechanistic Modelling

The principles of physics and biochemistry, as well as other basic rules of nature, provide the basis of mechanistic models. We can find the unknown model parameters—adsorption coefficients, diffusivity, or material properties—and calibrate the model with less experimental data. A wide range of real-world scenarios may benefit from the mechanistic modeling.

Statistical Parameters, Estimation

Different stastical parameters, 1. Measures of central tendency 2. Dispersion (also called Variability, Scatter, Spread) 3. Coefficient of Dispersion (COD) 4. Variance 5. Standard Deviation (SD) σ 6. Residuals 7. Factor Analysis 8. Absolute Error (AE) 9. Mean Absolute Error (MAE) 10. Percentage Error of Estimate (PE)

Research in the field of pharmacology relies heavily on statistical methods, which allow us to test hypotheses by describing the data using measures of central tendency and variance, such as the mean, median, standard deviation, confidence interval, and range. A parameter is a variable that is transmitted from one equation to another. It has a distinct statistical meaning. Values like these differ from statistics, which only provide information about subsets of a larger population, since they provide information about the whole population as a whole.

1. **Central Tendency:** Averages are another tem for measurements of central tendency. The degree to which the values are concentrated in the center of the distribution may be determined with their assistance. Some popular ways to find the middle ground are as follows: (i) Arithmetic mean, (ii) Median, (iii) Mode

   Mean: It is in the middle of the distribution and is the average of the data. The arithmetic mean is another name for it. For every given set of data, finding the mean is as easy as adding them all up and dividing by the collection size.

   Median: Finding the data point in the center of the sequence after sorting it from lowest to highest yields the middle value, which is the data set's median. As a measure of central tendency, the median takes a single number and shows how a collection of data clusters around that number. What this means is that it provides a means of describing the core of a dataset.

   Extreme Values have no effect on it.

   Mode: Most commonly occurring value and the mode is the most frequently occurring value in the data set. The mode is simple to compute and easily understood. Extreme levels have no affected whatsoever on mode. Even if the frequency distribution comprises class intervals with uneven magnitudes, the mode can still be easily found.

2. **Dispersion:** It refers to how much a distribution is compressed or stretched. The variance, standard deviation, and interquartile ranges are common illustrations of statistical dispersion.
3. **Coefficient of Dispersion (COD):** It is a unit-less measure of dispersion that characterizes the degree of dispersion with respect to the mean. $\boldsymbol{COD = \sigma / \mu * 100}$.
4. **Variance:** It is the expected squared variance of a random variable from its mean and generally measures the dispersion of a group of random values from the mean. It provides a numerical depiction of the data scatter by squaring the differences between each value in the set and the mean, dividing the sum of the squares by the total number of values in the set, and finally, displaying the results to the viewer.
5. **Standard Deviation (SD) Σ:** It is a metric for estimating how much a set of data values vary or are dispersed. It is a figure that indicates how a group's measurement deviates from the expected or mean value. When the standard deviation is low, the majority of the data are fairly near to the average; when it is large, the data are dispersed. The standard deviation gives the user a numerical representation of the data's spread.
6. **Residuals:** It is the discrepancy between the anticipated value (y') and the observed value (y) of the dependent variable. A residual is present for every data point. The residuals are all 0, both in terms of total and mean. $\boldsymbol{R = Observed\ Y\ value - Predicted\ Y\ value}$.
7. **Factor Analysis:** Collapsing a huge number of variables into a few interpretable underlying elements, it allows researchers to explore ideas that are not readily quantified directly by exploring variable connections for complicated concepts.
8. **Absolute Error:** This is the size of the discrepancy between the precise and approximate values. The absolute error, proportional to the precise value's size, is called the relative error.

$$Aabsolute\ Eerror = \boldsymbol{X\ measured - X\ actual}.$$

9. **Mean Absolute Error (MAE):** It is a quantity to measure how close forecasts or predictions are to the eventual outcomes. It is an average of the absolute errors. The simplest measure of forecast accuracy is MAE. The relative size of error is not always obvious.

10. **Percentage of Estimate (PE)**: It is the difference between the approximate and the exact values as a percentage of the exact value.

$$\% \, \boldsymbol{Error} = (\boldsymbol{Exact\ Value} - \boldsymbol{Approximate\ Value}) / \boldsymbol{Exact\ Value} \times \mathbf{100}.$$

Confidence Regions

An expanded version of a confidence interval that accounts for many dimensions is a confidence region. Representing the parameter values most likely to be true given the data, it is a collection of points in an n-dimensional space. The confidence zone is computed in a manner that, subject to several repetitions of the experiment, would, 95% of the time, include the actual parameter values.

Interpretation: The statistical concept of a confidence interval is the likelihood, on average, that a parameter representing a population will lie within a predetermined range of values. The likelihood that a parameter will lie between two values near the mean is shown by a confidence interval. The degree of certainty or uncertainty in a sampling process may be measured using confidence intervals. They are often built with 95% or 99% confidence levels. With a 95% level of certainty, you may say that any number inside the 95% confidence interval represents the population's actual mean. The sample mean (the center of the CI) will differ from one sample to the next as a result of inherent sampling variability.

Nonlinearity at the Optimum

When an independent variable does not have a direct connection with a dependent variable, the statistical concept of non-linearity is employed to characterize the situation. In nonlinear relationships, there are cases when the output does not respond linearly to changes in the inputs.

Sensitivity Analysis

The goal of a sensitivity analysis is to identify the many input sources of uncertainty and determine the relative contributions to numerical and non-numerical uncertainties in the output of a mathematical model or system. Similar ideas may be found in uncertainty analysis, which focuses more on measuring and communicating uncertainty. It is recommended to do sensitivity and uncertainty assessments together. There are many advantages to doing sensitivity analyses, which include recalculating results under different assumptions to determine the impact of a variable, including:

1. Testing the resilience of model or system results when faced with uncertainty.
2. Gaining deeper insight into the relationships between input and output variables within a model or system.
3. Reducing uncertainty by pinpointing model inputs that significantly contribute to output uncertainty, warranting focused attention for enhanced robustness, possibly through further research.
4. Finding inconsistencies or outliers in the model, often by discovering hidden relationships between parameters.
5. Fixing inputs that don't affect output or finding and removing unnecessary parts of the model structure might help make it more efficient.
6. Assisting modellers in conveying their findings to decision-makers in a way that is clear, concise, convincing, and easy to understand.
7. Identifying areas within the input factor space where the model output reaches its maximum, minimum, or fulfils certain optimal criteria, akin to optimization and Monte Carlo filtering.

When there are many parameters in a model, a main sensitivity test may help narrow the emphasis to the ones that matter most during calibration. It is possible to waste time on factors that are not sensitive if we do not take their sensitivity into account. We also want to find meaningful relationships between our observations, model inputs, predictions, and forecasts so that we can improve our models.

The choice of sensitivity analysis method typically depends on a variety of problem-specific constraints and settings.

Sensitivity Analysis Methods

Sensitivity analysis techniques encompass a wide array of approaches tailored to address various constraints. These methods are also differentiated by the nature of sensitivity measurement, encompassing variance decompositions, partial derivatives, or elementary effects. Here are some of the prominent sensitivity analysis methods:

1. **Derivative-based local method:** Finding the partial derivative of the model's output (Y) with respect to an input variable (Xi) is the key to this approach. Its goal, in a local setting, is to determine how little changes to input elements affect the output.

2. **Regression analysis:** Regression analysis, as it pertains to sensitivity analysis, comprises fitting a linear regression model to the model's response. Direct indications of sensitivity are provided by standardized regression coefficients. When a substantial coefficient of determination confirms that the model response is linear, regression analysis is most useful. Its advantages include simplicity and low computational overhead.
3. **Variance-based methods:** Included in this class are probabilistic methods that use probability distributions to depict input and output uncertainty. These techniques break down the total variation in output into its component parts, which may then be assigned to specific input factors or sets of variables. The degree to which an input variable affects the output is indicated by the amount of variation it causes.
4. **Variogram analysis of response surfaces (VARS):** Previous approaches to sensitivity analysis failed to account for the response surface's or model's output's spatially ordered structure in the parameter space (Y=f(X)). The VARS approach addresses this by employing directional variograms to comprehensively illustrate sensitivity information, accounting for both direction and perturbation scale concepts. By embracing the scale-dependent nature of sensitivity, VARS overcomes the scale-related challenges encountered by conventional methods.

   These sensitivity analysis approaches help to evaluate a model's behavior and performance in a comprehensive manner by providing several ways to analyze the links between input and output variables.

Optimal Design

When it comes to experimental design, there's a subfield called optimal designs that aims for perfection according to certain statistical standards. It was the Danish statistician Kirstine Smith who did the ground-breaking work in this field. When designing experiments, optimal designs are essential for estimating statistical models, as they allow for the estimate of parameters in an unbiased manner with minimal variation. To get the same degree of parameter accuracy as an ideal design, a larger number of experimental runs is required for a non-optimal design. Practically speaking, optimum experimental designs help bring down the cost of experiments. The determination of design optimality relies on the underlying statistical model and is evaluated based on a statistical criterion tied to the variance matrix of the estimator. The process of specifying an appropriate model and criterion function demands a sound understanding of statistical theory along with practical experience in experimental design.

Among the many requirements for design optimization, a popular strategy is to choose time points so that the dispersion of parameter estimates, which is estimated at the optimal point by the inverse of the Fisher information matrix (FIM), is minimized. Finding the best times to sample in three-, eight-, or twelve-sample trials is a common research topic, and one prominent approach is D-optimal design (where D stands for determinant). The main idea is to create a large, fake sample of parameters with appropriately dispersed values. Optimal time selection is defined as maximizing the FIM determinant for all possible values of the parameters. This leads to the determination of a set of optimal sampling times corresponding to each parameter value. Subsequently, a histogram is constructed to visualize the frequency of optimal sampling time choices. This empirical distribution guides the selection of the most suitable sampling times for subsequent experiments.

Optimal designs offer distinct advantages over sub-optimal experimental designs, including the following key benefits:

1. **Cost Reduction:** Optimal designs contribute to lowering experimentation costs by enabling statistical model estimation with a reduced number of experimental runs.
2. **Versatility:** Optimal designs are flexible and adaptable, accommodating diverse factors such as process, mixture, and discrete factors.
3. **Constrained Design-Space:** When the design-space is small or restricted, optimal designs may be used, particularly when certain factor-settings are not feasible because of safety concerns or other constraints.

In summary, optimal experimental designs significantly enhance the efficiency and effectiveness of experimental processes by enabling accurate parameter estimation with minimal resource expenditure. Their versatility and adaptability make them valuable tools for various types of experimental scenarios and constraints.

Different Criterion of Optimal Design

It is important to compare the designs' performance across several optimality criteria, and picking the right one takes some consideration.

A-optimality ("average" or trace): The A-optimality criterion minimizes the trace of the inverse of the information matrix and is one of the criteria. Regression coefficient estimates with the least average variance are those that meet this requirement.

C-optimality: For a set of linear parameters in the model, this criteria seeks to minimize the variance of the best linear unbiased estimator.

D-optimality (determinant): A well-liked metric is D-optimality, which aims to reduce the absolute value of $X'X^{-1}$ or, in other words, maximize the determinant of the design's information matrix X'X. The goal of these criteria is to maximize the parameter estimates' differential Shannon information content.

E-optimality (eigenvalue): Another design is E-optimality, which maximizes the minimum eigenvalue of the information matrix.

T-optimality: This criterion maximizes the trace of the information matrix. Other optimality-criteria are concerned with the variance of predictions is

G-optimality: The G-optimality criteria aims to minimize the greatest entry in the diagonal of the hat matrix $X\,(X'X)^{-1}X'$, and it is widely used. The worst-case scenario for the expected values is reduced as a result.

I-optimality (integrated): Optimality, which aims to reduce the average prediction variance across the design space, is a second criteria on prediction variance.

V-optimality (variance): Thirdly, V-optimality attempts to minimize the average prediction variance across a collection of m particular points, which is a measure of prediction variance.

Implementation

Books and software libraries include catalogs of ideal designs. Plus, there are features in popular statistical packages like R and SAS that allow users to optimize designs according to their specifications. A model for the design and an optimality criteria must be specified by the experimenter before the approach may calculate an optimal design. Additional statistical theory and experience with experimental design are prerequisites for some more advanced optimum design subjects.

Practical considerations

More theoretical understanding of statistics and hands-on experience with experiment design is required for certain more sophisticated optimum design issues.

Based on the model and optimality criteria, top-notch statistical software offers either built-in libraries of optimal designs or iterative ways to generate nearly optimum designs. A predefined optimality criteria is available, or users may code their own.

1. Atkinson, Donev, and Tobias document these three benefits (of optimum designs) in the textbook.
2. In optimization theory, these kinds of criteria are known as objective functions.
3. Fundamental notions in statistical theory include the Fisher information functional and other "information" functions.

Population Modeling

Modeling plays a pivotal role in the realm of drug development, particularly in the intricate process of population modeling, which necessitates robust underlying methodologies to ensure data accuracy, suitable computational platforms, sufficient resources, and effective communication. Despite the resource investment required, this approach can lead to time and cost savings by creating a platform to consolidate all information pertaining to novel therapeutic agents. Models lay the groundwork for explaining and understanding the time course of drug exposure and response following the administration of different formulations or dosages to people. Drug clearance and distribution volume are two critical characteristics that might be estimated with their help. Consistency between studies or patient groups may be ensured by constructing population models with relatively few data from each subject. The resulting parameter estimations can then be compared with past evaluations. Additionally, these estimates can be juxtaposed against data related to other drugs in the same therapeutic category, aiding in evaluating the developmental prospects of new therapeutic agents.

Population modeling assessment boils down to developing a mathematical function that can represent a drug's pharmacological time course over a range of clinical trial dosages. The importance of careful dosage selection and regimen planning in turning medications from dangerous substances into useful therapeutic tools has been highlighted by Atkinson and Lalonde. Hence, modeling and simulation have become essential tools for integrating information, understanding, and processes to direct prudent choices about medication use and development. There are several areas of drug research that rely heavily on modeling and simulation; Figure 1 provides a brief summary of these areas. Predicting exposure and response trajectories under different dosage regimens is made easier with the use of appropriate models.

An important step in this development is the broad use of population modeling methods, which provide a structure for measuring and understanding the variability in pharmacological exposure and response. Through the use of population modeling, the relationships between a person's physiological characteristics and their reported drug exposure or reaction may be better understood and described. The idea was first proposed by Sheiner et al. in 1972 to deal with sparse pharmacokinetic (PK) data captured during therapeutic drug monitoring, but it has since been extended to include models that link drug concentration to response (pharmacodynamic or PD). Consequently, modeling has become an essential tool in the process of developing drugs.

Two methods were previously used to estimate population parameters: one was the "naive pooled approach," which fitted data from all individuals simultaneously and ignored individual differences, and the other was the "two-stage approach," which fitted data from each individual separately and then aggregated their parameter estimates to produce population parameters. Dosage compliance, missing data, and other inaccuracies may amplify the problems with both methodologies, making it much more difficult to get accurate parameter estimations. By eliminating the drawbacks of previous methods, Sheiner et al. were able to estimate population mean parameters, between-subject variability (BSV), and the effects of covariates that shed light on drug exposure variability using sparse data from many subjects. By using this method, standard errors could be generated, which allowed for an evaluation of parameter accuracy.

The phrase "population PK" may make it sound like individual patients aren't important, but the explanation of variability highlights how important they are in population models. Each person's data helps find patterns, such how drug exposure increases with age or how weight changes, and then we can estimate population features based on those trends. Pharmacometrics harnesses these insights to enhance our understanding of mechanisms, guide initial dose selection for testing, tailor or personalize dosages for patient subpopulations, and evaluate study design appropriateness.

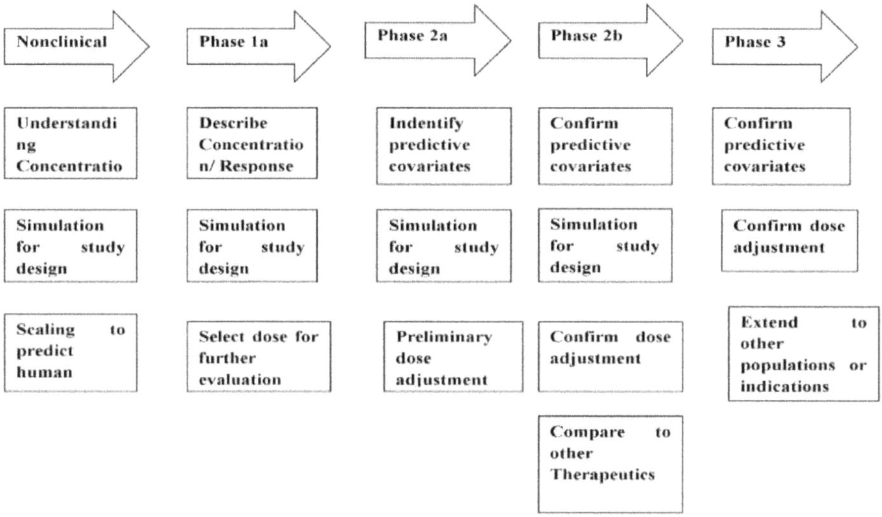

FIGURE 1 Brief outline of some areas in which modeling and simulation are commonly employed during drug development.

Quality by Design in Pharmaceutical Development

Starting with established goals, quality by design (QbD) places an emphasis on item and cycle knowledge and controls based on solid science and the quality risk board (ICH Q8), and it is an effective method for dealing with product improvement. The concept of Quality by Configuration was first proposed by Joseph M. Juran. It is possible to combine product and process knowledge acquired throughout development by building needed qualities from data process knowledge. The main objective of QbD is to achieve the quality products are

1. Ensure better design of product with fewer problems.
2. Continuous improvement.
3. Better understanding of the process.
4. Maximize productivity in production while decreasing expenses, project rejections, and waste.
5. Empowerment of technical staff.
6. Minimize deviations and costly investigations.
7. Eliminate batch failures.
8. Benefits of QBD for Industry.

Tools Applied in QBD Approach

Design of Experiment (DoE): If you want the most dramatic results from your lead testing, this is the way to go. Minitab and Statistica are examples of programming tools that may be used to conduct a DoE. This allows for the screening of many parameters with few experimentation in order to determine the significant ones. The primary goal of these instruments is to identify basic effects, rather than the impacts of cooperation. Two ways exist for doing a DoE: screening methods using a fragmented factorial design or a Placket-Burman test. Alternatively, in the second approach, optimization, main and interaction effects are investigated using mixture designs, surface response methodologies (such as Central composite and Box-Behnken), and complete factorial designs.

Applications of Quality-By-Design

In Quality Profiling and Optimization of Drug Products

With advancements in technology and the development of modern production tools, the industry has seen improvements in quality and cost reduction due to vast research, technological developments and the introduction of innovative manufacturing gear. Quality by Design (QbD) is quickly becoming the approach of choice in pharmaceutical research. It places a focus on understanding the product and the process, which in turn prioritizes scientific rigor and quality risk management. The idea of Quality by Design was first proposed by Joseph M. Juran. Adherence to the specifications outlined in ICH Q 8 and Q 9 is critical for risk assessment and the delivery of high-quality products. Design of Experiment (DoE) is an essential aspect of Quality by Design (QbD) and is a methodical approach to conducting experiments using software like Statistica, Minitab, and statease in order to maximize output. There are two approaches to experimental design. DoE is used in the screening and optimising different phases of formulation development. Screening is used to uncover important characteristics among many candidates with a minimum of experimentation. The primary goal of both the Placket-Burman and the fractional factorial design is to single out the most important effects. However, in optimisation, complete factorial designs, surface response techniques (such as Central composite, Box-Behnken), and mixed designs are often regarded to be carried out. These designing experiments are used only when certain aspects that appear to be contributing in process or formulation have been identified. During QbD approach for optimization study of different parameters are essential.

To validate the medicinal product's quality profile and minimize interactions among the input variables for optimization, pharmaceutical researchers often use AI features such as Quality by Design (QbD) and Design of Experiment (DoE). In a study conducted by Prusty et al. (2012), an extended-release matrix tablet containing benedipine hydrochloride was developed. The tablet was designed using the Box-Behnken Design Response Surface Methodology to Study Optimized Formulation Variables on the Drug Release Pattern. The researchers used one-way ANOVA to statistically analyze the tablets, and the quadratic response surface methodology (BBD) was used to predict the optimal levels of these factors for extending the drug's release. A number of mathematical models were used to kinetically assess the in vitro drug release data. Using the Quality by Design (QbD) approach in pharmaceutical goods allows for the study of many crucial criteria, including

i. ***Target product profile (TPP) and Quality Target Product profile (QTPP)***

   It reveals the high standards of the drug's quality that guarantee its effectiveness and safety. Dosage form, administration method, dose strength, pharmacokinetics, and stability are all important details to include in a product profile. Because it is organized according to the most significant parts of the drug's label and emphasizes the product's intended performance features in connection to the patient's demand, the TPP is a patient- and labeling-centered concept. Similarly, when it comes to issues of scientific security, QTPP offers a numerical alternative. The Quality Target Product Profile (QTPP) should only include patient-related efficacy that may be used to develop and optimize a formulation and production process. "Identity," "assay," "dosage form," "purity," and "stability" are some of the labeling problems with QTPP materials. Among the many potential quality aspects of a pharmaceutical product are its identity, assay, content homogeneity, microbiological restrictions, residual solvents, degradation products, drug release, and moisture content.

ii. ***Critical Quality Attributes (CQAs) and Critical Material Attributes (CMAs)***

   CQAs are qualities (physical, chemical, biological, or microbiological) that should fall within acceptable ranges to ensure the product meets quality standards. CMAs are characteristics of raw materials that must remain within predetermined parameters in order to produce consistent, high-quality drug compounds, excipients, or intermediates.

iii. Critical Process Parameters (CPP)

These characteristics are production process variables that may affect finished product CQAs. Performing risk assessments at various points in the product lifecycle helps identify process characteristics and Critical Manufacturing Attributes (CMAs). The proven collection of input variables and process parameters that ensure quality is called the Design Space.

iv. Design Space

A pharmaceutical's design space (DS) is the variety of potential material and process circumstances that nevertheless guarantees high quality. This is the proven, multi-factor combination of input factors (such as material qualities) and process parameters that ensures quality.

v. Failure Mode Effects Analysis (FMEA)

Failure mode and effect analysis (FMEA) is a method for evaluating risk that involves analyzing the probability functions of an event's severity, occurrence, and detectability.

vi. PAT (Process Analytical Technology)

According to the Food and Drug Administration (FDA), Process Analytical Technology (PAT) is "a mechanism for designing, analysing, and controlling pharmaceutical manufacturing processes by measuring critical process parameters that affect critical quality attributes of an active pharmaceutical ingredient (API) during manufacturing."

In order to manage the drug development process more effectively, artificial intelligence approaches that use Machine Learning techniques have become essential. These models employ real-world information to inform their forecasts and design decisions, boosting output, uniformity, and quality in the process. The use of machine learning in the pharmaceutical industry presents a great chance to create new, more effective drug compositions. In conclusion, the adoption of Quality by Design (QbD) principles, combined with machine learning and advanced technology, is transforming the pharmaceutical industry. With a focus on product and process understanding, risk management, and continuous improvement, QbD is paving the way for safer and more effective drug formulations in a cost-effective manner.

ICH Q8 Guideline

Quality by Design (QbD) is based on the guiding concepts laid forth in the ICH quality standards, which include a science-based approach to product creation, risk assessment, a lifecycle approach, and method design. A few notable documents that embody these ideas include the ICH Q8 Pharmaceutical Development, the ICH Q9 Quality Risk Management, and the ICH Q10 Pharmaceutical Quality System.

The International Conference on Harmonization (ICH) Q8 standard established the idea of Quality by Design (QbD). Process control based on strong scientific principles and quality risk management are the tenets of this methodical approach, which begins with established goals and places an emphasis on product and process understanding. In particular, ICH Q8 highlights the need of 'quality by design' being seamlessly integrated into the drug's lifetime and pharmaceutical development. By committing to ICH Q8 compliance, organizations may embed consistent operational quality throughout their processes, making quality a top priority.

Important components, such as medicinal ingredients, excipients, container sealing mechanisms, and production procedures, that substantially impact product quality are identified under the purview of ICH Q8. Determining these crucial characteristics and justifying control measures are emphasized in the guideline. Proposed methods for efficient allocation of design space include experimental designs, Process Analytical Technology (PAT), previous knowledge, and quality risk management concepts.

Process Analytical Technology, or PAT for short, is essential to the Quality by Design methodology. It entails taking quick readings of important performance and quality indicators while production is underway. As a result, the quality of the finished product may be more reliably assured. Importantly, Pfizer was an early adopter of QbD and PAT practices.

The Quality Target Product Profile (QTPP) is an essential part of Quality by Design (QbD) as it provides an overview of a drug's quality features in the future, taking safety and effectiveness into account. Part of this process is figuring out what the product's most important process parameters (CPPs) and quality characteristics are. Product quality attributes (CQAs) are those that guarantee the product meets the specified standards, while process parameters (CPPs) have an immediate effect on CQAs.

Drug Substances

The medication substance's physicochemical and biological characteristics may impact the product's performance and its manufacturability. Solubility, water content, particle size, crystal characteristics, biological activity, and permeability are some of the desirable qualities that should be investigated.

Excipients

Discuss the selected excipients and their concentrations in light of how they will affect the drug product's performance and manufacturability. The drug substance's compatibility with the chosen excipients must be evaluated. If the product contains multiple drug substances, the compatibility between these substances should also be assessed.

Formulation Development

A description of the formulation development process should be provided. The process begins with the formulation's conceptualization and continues until its final design, during which time the qualities essential to the drug product's quality are identified. All clinical formulations should be linked to the proposed commercial formulation by comparative in vitro or in vivo investigations, such as dissolution or bioequivalence. If the correlations work, it will be easier to choose suitable dissolution acceptability criteria and, after making adjustments to the product or manufacturing process, there may be less need for further bioequivalence studies.

Container and Closure System

It is important to analyze potential interactions between the product, container, and label when choosing the container closure system for the commercial product. This includes studying the right reasons for choosing the materials for main and secondary packing.

Microbiological Attributes

It is important to consider the antibacterial properties of specific items as well as the efficacy of preservative systems in products that include these substances. Verifying that the container closure method effectively prevents microbiological contamination is essential for sterile items. Making sure the concentration maintains the necessary effectiveness throughout the product's planned shelf life, the rationale for the lowest stated concentration of antimicrobial preservative should revolve on safety and efficacy.

Compatibility

It is important to address concerns like precipitation and stability when discussing the therapeutic product's compatibility with reconstitution diluents. The data should include the suggested in-use duration, the ideal temperature for storage, and the most probable concentration extremes. Also, things to think about when diluting or admixing items before administration (such putting the product in big volume infusion containers) should be taken into account.

Regulatory and Industry Views On QBD

Customer happiness with service, product, and process is an indicator of quality. Timely, low-value, flawless, and dependable performance is what the client is requesting. There are two approaches to ensure customer satisfaction: offering alternatives and ensuring the product is free from defects. A rise in product quality is on the horizon as a result of new regulatory initiatives.

FDA perspective

Pharmaceutical firms were requested by the US Food and Drug Administration (FDA) in 2005 to provide chemistry, manufacturing, and controls (CMC) information in their New Drug Applications (NDAs) that demonstrated the adoption of Quality by Design (QbD). Understanding the product's essential quality characteristics (CQAs) and developing a manufacturing process that can reliably create products that fulfill those CQAs are the primary goals of quality by design (QbD), a risk-based approach to pharmaceutical development.

The FDA's decision to adopt QbD was based on several factors, including:

1. The increasing complexity of pharmaceutical manufacturing processes.
2. The need to improve the quality and consistency of pharmaceutical products.
3. The desire to reduce the number of manufacturing changes that require regulatory approval.

   Despite its complexity and difficulty, Quality by Design (QbD) offers great promise for enhancing the security and efficacy of pharmaceuticals.

The key elements of QbD include:

1. Defining the product's CQAs: The first step in QbD is to identify the CQAs of the product. Important to the product's security and usefulness are these features.
2. Understanding the manufacturing process: The next step is to understand the manufacturing process that will be used to produce the product. This includes understanding the factors that can affect the CQAs of the product.
3. Designing a robust manufacturing process: Designing a strong manufacturing process requires first understanding the product and process CQAs. This is a process that is designed to consistently produce products that meet the CQAs, even in the face of variations in the raw materials or manufacturing conditions.
4. Implementing a risk-based approach to quality: A risk-based approach to quality is also an integral part of QbD. This entails finding potential threats to the product's quality, evaluating them, and then adopting measures to lessen their impact.

QbD is a relatively new approach to pharmaceutical development, but it is gaining widespread acceptance in the industry. The FDA has stated that QbD is the preferred approach to pharmaceutical development, and many pharmaceutical companies are now adopting QbD principles.

With the arrival of 2005 came the time to adopt QbD for a more systematic approach, and the USFDA requested that some companies submit their CMC in QbD format. The QbD approach is built upon question basis review (QbR).

Regulatory Challenges and Inspection

According to Anastasia G. Lolas and Anurag S. Rathore, "In a QbD concept, the regulatory burden is less because there are wider ranges and limits based on product and process understanding. Changes within these ranges and limits do not require prior approval."

The system-based methodology and CDER's Compliance Program "Inspection of Licensed Biological Therapeutic Drug Products" have traditionally been used for inspections by the FDA. Nevertheless, in this case of QbD being required, the FDA inspection team will evaluate the application-described process design's execution and efficacy, as well as the transfer of knowledge and risk management from development to production. The efficacy of the quality system in ensuring consistent product quality, managing deviations, improving processes, implementing changes to control procedures, and managing knowledge and risk throughout the product lifecycle will also be assessed during the inspection.

There will be no change to the previously conducted inspections of supplier management, raw material screening, and facility and equipment qualification and maintenance. On the other hand, we will emphasize the programs that show consistency and robustness in design, testing, and monitoring. Programs for design, testing, and monitoring that show consistency and robustness would be commended.

Because there is a unit broader range and limitations supported product and technique comprehension in a QbD concept, the restricting load is reduced. These ranges and restrictions may be changed without prior permission.

The CDER's Compliance Program "Inspection of accredited Biological Therapeutic Drug Products" and the FDA's system-based approach are the usual means of conducting inspections. But the question that comes up in this context is how the investigation can guarantee the location of any QbD that is outsourced. When the FDA examines a QbD concept during pre-license or preapproval inspections, they can see how well the method design is implemented and how well data and risk management are transferred from development to production. In terms of data and risk management, method improvements, modification management, consistent product quality, and deviation management, the standard system may be examined and assessed for its efficacy throughout the product lifespan. Due to its accidental nature, the review of abilities and instrumentality qualifications and maintenance, as well as raw material screening and provider management, are same. However, programs that show lustiness and consistency in their design, testing, and observation would be commended.

When it comes to implementing QbD, most pharmaceutical companies believe that easier guidance is required. Companies sought the federal agency's elucidation on QbD jargon, appropriate methods, criteria for selecting and deselecting CQAs, standards for determining if controls are adequate, and criteria for replacing analytical techniques. The ten most significant obstacles to QbD adoption are as follows. At various stages of adoption, these obstacles are assessed in relation to other medication kinds.

The first four challenges occur at companies and these are

1. Internal placement refers to the separation of many practical domains, such as research and development (R&D) and production (or quality and regulation).
2. Disbelief in the business case, or the fact that many questions remain unanswered about the timing and budgetary requirements for implementing QbD.
3. Inadequate tools for the job (such as problem management software or a lack of knowledge about the consequences of critical quality attribute [CQA]).
4. Contract manufacturers and suppliers are becoming more important in QbD implementation, so how can we ensure their alignment?

The next six challenges are directly associated with the regulative authority:

1. Discordant handling of QbD by various administrative bodies
2. No real direction for the company
3. Authorities are ill-prepared to deal with QbD applications.
4. A method to get regulatory benefits The information that is currently being supplied does not instill trust.
5. The failure of global regulatory agencies to work together
6. Current interaction with corporations isn't causative to QbD.

All parties agree that the only way to overcome the obstacles and problems with QbD implementation is for businesses and regulatory agencies to have an economical discourse.

Bibliography

1. Atkinson A.J., Jr, &, Lalonde R.L. Introduction of quantitative methods in pharmacology and clinical pharmacology: a historical overview. *Clin. Pharmacol. Ther.* 2007; 82:3–6. [PubMed] [Google Scholar]
2. Box G.E.P., &, Draper N.R. John Wiley & Sons, Inc. New York; 1986. *Empirical Model-building and Response Surfaces*. [Google Scholar]
3. Cobelli C, Foster D, Toffolo G. Kluwer Academic/Plenum Publishers, New York; 2000. *Tracer Kinetics in Biomedical Research: From Data to Model*. [Google Scholar
4. Drakulich, A. Critical challenges to implementing QbD: AQ and A with FDA. Pharm Technol 2009; 33: 90-4.

5. Hull C.J., &, McLeod K. Pharmacokinetic analysis using an electrical analogue. *Br. J. Anaesth.* 1976; 48: 677–686. [PubMed] [Google Scholar]
6. Jain S. Quality by design (QbD): A comprehensive understanding of implementation and challenges in pharmaceutical development. Int J Pharm Pharm Sci 2013; 6: 29-35.
7. Moheb MN. Implementation of Quality by Design (QbD) Current Perspectives on Opportunities and Challenges Topic Introduction and ICH Update, Office of New Drug Quality Assessment OPS/ CDER/ FDA Advisory Committee for Pharmaceutical Science and Clinical Pharmacology; 2014.
8. Nikkelen E., van Meurs W.L., &, Ohrn M.A. Hydraulic analog for simultaneous representation of pharmacokinetics and pharmacodynamics: application to vecuronium. *J. Clin. Monit. Comput.* 1998; 14:329–337. [PubMed] [Google Scholar]
9. Sheiner L.B. The population approach to pharmacokinetic data analysis: rationale and standard data analysis methods. *Drug Metab. Rev.* 1984; 15:153–171. [PubMed] [Google Scholar]
10. Sheiner L.B., &, Beal S.L. Evaluation of methods for estimating population pharmacokinetics parameters. I. Michaelis-Menten model: routine clinical pharmacokinetic data. *J. Pharmacokinet. Biopharm.* 1980; 8: 553–571. [PubMed] [Google Scholar]
11. Sheiner L.B., Rosenberg B., &, Melmon K.L. Modelling of individual pharmacokinetics for computer-aided drug dosage. *Comput. Biomed. Res.* 1972; 5: 411–459. [PubMed] [Google Scholar]
12. Stanski D.R., &, Maitre P.O. Population pharmacokinetics and pharmacodynamics of thiopental: the effect of age revisited. *Anesthesiology.* 1990; 72: 412–422. [PubMed] [Google Scholar]
13. Whiting B., Kelman A.W., &, Grevel J. Population pharmacokinetics. Theory and clinical application. *Clin. Pharmacokinet.* 1986; 11: 387–401. [PubMed] [Google Scholar]

UNIT II

Computational Modelling of Drug Disposition Simulation Modelling

Simulation modeling involves a computational representation of a system, incorporating numerous variables that define its characteristics. The process of simulation entails adjusting these variables individually or in combination, observing the resulting outcomes. Through computer modeling, researchers can simulate a multitude of experiments efficiently. It emulates the functioning of real-world processes or systems over time, generating artificial histories of systems and extracting insights from them. Assuming logical, symbolic, and mathematical links between different parts of the system is fundamental to this method.

Importance of Simulation Modeling

1. It makes it easier to examine and experiment with the inner workings of complicated systems and subsystems.
2. Informational, organizational, and environmental changes may be represented and observed via simulation of the model's behavior.
3. Important information is uncovered that may be used to propose improvements to the system being studied.
4. Finding important variables and their interactions in a simulation becomes feasible by changing inputs and seeing outcomes.
5. Simulation serves as a tool to reinforce analytical solution methodologies.
6. It can be used to verify analytical solutions.
7. Simulation aids in experimenting with new designs or policies before implementation, providing a preparedness mechanism.
8. Designed for training purposes, simulation allows for learning without the disruptions and costs associated with on-the-job training.

9. In the context of modern complex systems, simulations are essential to understanding intricate interactions.
10. Changing simulation inputs and observing outputs provides insight into key variables and their interactions.
11. Simulation can also be used to validate analytical solutions.

Empirical Classical Compartmental Model

Subsequent to administration to the gastrointestinal tract, the traditional compartmental model predicts how much of the medication will be absorbed into the bloodstream as a function of the absorption rate constant (ka). This process is controlled by a constant called the elimination rate (ke). Absorption is usually described as a single first-order process in this approach. A lag period is often included in empirical absorption models that assume first-order or zero-order absorption kinetics. Simple compartmental modeling of plasma concentration-time profiles may be used to estimate absorption rate constants.

Importance of Models in Drug Disposition

Drug Absorption

The simplicity and high rate of patient compliance make oral administration the favored mode of medication delivery. Oral medication absorption, which mostly occurs in the human gut, is the primary focus of in silico methods. Drug solubility and intestinal permeability interact to determine bioavailability and absorption.

Drug Distribution

A drug's pharmacokinetic profile is greatly impacted by its distribution. Volumn of distribution (VD), plasma-protein binding (PPB), and blood-brain barrier (BBB) permeability are some of the physiochemical and structural features that determine the degree to which a medicine is distributed. Using VD in conjunction with drug clearance allows for the prediction of drug half-life by reflecting the drug's partitioning between plasma and tissue. Although predicting VD solely based on computed descriptors is under development due to limited in vivo data and complex processes, progress has been made in this direction. Using two in vitro physicochemical factors, Lombardo and colleagues provide a method for predicting VD for both basic and neutral substances. This model has expanded with additional data, improving accuracy in predicting VD.

Types of Computational Modeling

1. Molecular docking (Lock & key)
2. Pharmacophore (2D & 3D)

Molecular Docking

In order to better comprehend how tiny molecules behave at the binding site of target proteins and to shed light on basic biological reactions, the molecular docking method may be used to simulate the atomic-level interaction between two molecules. Generally there are two distinct forms of docking;

Rigid Docking

Docking Brackets The molecules in the stiff molecule docking issue are inherently immobile and unable to undergo any kind of spatial shape change once docked. Taking into consideration that the compounds are rigid, our goal is to find a three-dimensional arrangement of one of them that maximizes the degree to which it matches the other compounds according to a scoring system's characteristics. The creation of the ligands' conformations is not dependent on their ability to bind to receptors.

Flexible Docking

Docking Systems with Adaptability As stiff objects, molecules may undergo changes in spatial form when docking, which is the root of the rigid molecule docking issue. We assess molecular flexibility in tandem with transformation to find confirmations for the receptor and ligand molecules in their complex states.

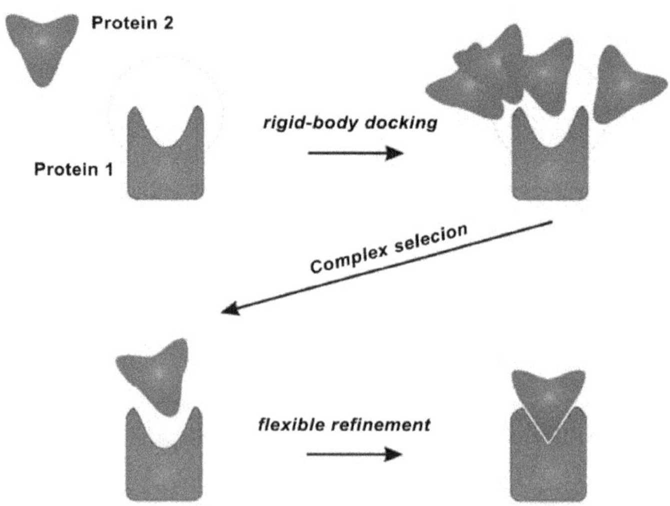

FIGURE 1 Representation of Different types of Molecular Docking.

Pharmacophore

The computational method of pharmacophore modeling employs structural and ligand-based techniques and finds use in a wide range of computational biological applications. Many CADD tasks may benefit from pharmacophore modeling. Both structure-based and ligand-based approaches exist. If we know the residues in a protein's binding pocket in a structure-based pharmacophore, we can use those features to search a database for potential ligands. However, in ligand-base pharmacophore modeling, we can either build a pharmacophore based on the characteristics of the protein's natural ligand to find compounds with a stronger affinity for the protein's active site than the ligand itself, or we can use the best compound that has been reported to be an inhibitor for that protein to build our pharmacophore.

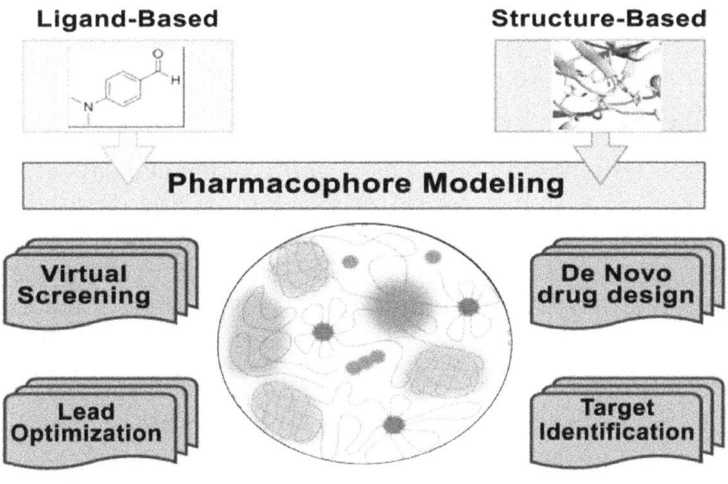

FIGURE 2 Representation of Pharmacophore modelling.

Modeling Techniques Pharmaceutical Parameter Consider in Drug Absorption

1. Lipophilicity or Calculation of log p value

Because it affects a compound's solubility, permeability, potency, selectivity, and promiscuity, lipophilicity is a crucial metric in the drug development process. The logarithm of the concentration of a chemical in an equilibrium mixture of octanol and water, expressed as Po/w, is a common way to measure the lipophilicity of organic compounds. Pharmaceutical companies can't maximize the pharmacodynamic and pharmacokinetic features of hits and leads without first predicting log P. Ab initio approaches based on molecular simulation, substructure-based methods, and property-based methods are the three main categories into which the existing methods for determining log P fall. Thermodynamic integration-based molecular dynamics simulations were used to quantify the absolute solvation Gibbs free energies in various phases at constant temperature (T) and pressure (P), which were used to build ab initio techniques for log P prediction.

$$\mathbf{Log\ P^{o/w} = \Delta G^{oct}{}_{solv} - \Delta G^{w}{}_{solv}/2.303RT}$$

Where $\Delta G^{oct}{}_{solv}$ is the solvation Gibbs free energies of compounds in water-saturated octanol,

$\Delta G^{w}{}_{solv}$ is the solvation Gibbs free energies of compounds in water,

R is the molar gas constant and

T is the temperature (298 K).

Therefore, obtaining the salvation free energies of compounds in each phase is the key step in the log P calculation.

2. Solubility

A pivotal determinant impacting drug bioavailability is aqueous solubility. For a drug to be absorbed, it must first dissolve in water and then traverse biological membranes. Sublimation from crystal to vapour and then to solution are the two stages of the dissolution process that a thermodynamic cycle uses to predict solubility. We may thus state the connection as between intrinsic solubility (S0) and the total change in Gibbs free energy.

$$\mathbf{\Delta G^{*}_{sol} = \Delta G^{*}_{sub} + \Delta G^{*}_{sol} - RT\ ln\ S_0V_m,}$$

ΔG^{*}_{sol} is the Gibbs free energy for solution,

ΔG^{*}_{sub} is the Gibbs free energy for sublimation,

ΔG^{*}_{solv} is the Gibbs free energy for solvation,

R is the molar gas constant

T is the temperature

Thermodynamic cycle for the transfer from crystal to vapour and then to solution

3. Ionization Constant

The ionization constant, measured as pKa, is a crucial parameter influencing various molecular properties. At physiological pH, the ionized state of a medication has a significant impact on its diffusion and distribution. Ionized species are polar and soluble in water, while neutral species are more lipophilic. Log D, an expansion of log

P, takes into consideration the impact of ionization on the octanol-water partition coefficients and takes into consideration all possible configurations of the chemical. The majority of the oral medications that have been discovered either have invisible groups, always include ionized components, or come in different forms like salts. In order to get pKa data early on in the research and development process, high-throughput pKa screening and prediction techniques were created.

4. **ADME Prediction model**

   Drug interaction with the human body involves a dual process of drug effects and body disposal. ADME properties are pivotal factors determining a compound's drug ability. ADME prediction models simplify this complex process by focusing on key components or single processes. Plasma protein binding (PPB), blood-brain barrier (BBB) penetration, transporter interactions, and metabolic prediction, distribution, and intestinal absorption are all part of these models. Such models aid drug discovery by evaluating efficacy, selectivity, ADME, and toxicity, thus reducing attrition rates.

5. **Human Intestinal Absorption Model (HIA)**

   HIA predicts total absorption at specified dose levels, identifies limiting factors, assesses pH-dependent solubility, and forecasts absorption from different segments of the gastrointestinal tract. It provides valuable insight into absorption over time.

In Drug Distribution

1. **Plasma Protien Binding**

   Consistent rates of drug binding to plasma proteins may reduce bioavailability and cause undesirable drug-drug interactions (DDIs). Predicting binding rates and making the required adjustments to problematic drug candidates becomes crucial, as a result. When looking for compounds with a high binding affinity to human serum albumin (HSA), drug discovery researchers often use high-performance liquid chromatography (HPLC).

   But there are limits to this method. In the first place, crystallographic investigations have shown that there are many possible locations for ligand binding. Furthermore, the ever-changing character of HSA cannot be adequately captured by an immobilized column. A more all-encompassing approach to these problems might be to merge computational docking with MD analysis and HPLC data mining algorithms. For example, compounds may be classified according to their structural properties, or docking studies can determine which precise PPB site a chemical would bind to. It is possible to predict the compound-to-docking site binding affinity using docking or MD simulation methods in conjunction with HPLC data.

Numerous in silico models have been put forth, primarily focusing on two essential aspects:

1. Binding rate and affinity, directly assessing how strongly a drug attaches to HSA.
2. Binding sites and poses, providing valuable insights for potential structural modifications.

Characteristics of small molecules can be directly utilized for predicting binding sites and affinities, leading to the development of ligand-based HSA binding models. The five most important structural characteristics impacting PPB have been identified using the Plasma Protein Interaction Quantitative Structure-Activity Relationship (PPI-QSAR) model. In addition, this model has confirmed and predicted interactions between HSA and its ligands by using receptor-based approaches such MD simulation and docking. The binding constant is determined by for a certain concentration of drug-binding sites, assuming that each HAS molecule has a single binding site.

$$\text{Log } K_{HSA} = \log((t - t_0)/t_0)$$

Where t and t_0 are the retention times of the drug

2. Blood Brain Barrier

The tiny vascular endothelial cell layer that separates the brain from the circulation is known as the blood-brain barrier (BBB). The need for strong penetration in medications targeting the central nervous system (CNS) makes this distinction all the more important. Contrarily, in order to prevent unwanted side effects, it is crucial to minimize BBB penetration for non-CNS medications. There are a lot of moving parts in the complicated systems that allow chemicals to cross the BBB.

Passive diffusion and several catalyzed transport processes allow compounds to enter or leave the brain across the blood-brain barrier (BBB). Both receptor-mediated transcytosis and carrier-mediated transport are examples of such systems. The very complicated structure of BBB makes it difficult to evaluate its penetration. To determine if new chemicals have the ability to cross the blood-brain barrier, many methods have been devised. The gold standard for assessing BBB penetration, which includes both non-invasive and invasive methods, is in vivo brain uptake tests.

The rate and amount of brain permeation are key concepts utilized to estimate BBB permeability within in vivo investigations. The logarithm of the permeable-surface area product (log PS) and the logarithm of the brain/blood partitioning ratio at steady state (log BB) are the corresponding representations of these ideas. Although log BB is often used to measure BBB penetration, it only shows the total brain drug concentration and not the free drug concentration. A better indication would be log PS, as it directly measures BBB apparent permeability while accounting for the effects of plasma protein binding (PPB) and non-specific brain binding. Although in vivo models are important, they are often expensive and have poor throughput. A dearth of in vitro models that faithfully reproduce the in vivo BBB's characteristics is another issue. This highlights the need of developing more effective and efficient ways to measure the permeability of chemicals across the BBB and the difficulties of researching BBB penetration.

In Drug Metabolism

In the realm of drug metabolism, prediction models play a pivotal role by focusing on interactions between enzymes and xenobiotic, liver clearance, site of metabolism (SOM), and metabolite predictions. These models offer insights into drug metabolism, guiding drug discovery efforts. The identification of SOM aids in predicting vulnerable areas on xenobiotic molecules. Moreover, there are predictive models designed to anticipate all potential metabolites for a given xenobiotic compound.

Membrane Transporter

Membrane transporters are integral components in transmembrane processes that significantly impact the transfer of drugs. Drug distribution is greatly influenced by active transporters in particular. Unfortunately, our current level of knowledge about the processes behind active transporter effects limits their incorporation into models. Transporters with diverse characteristics and roles have attracted extensive attention. These include P-glycoprotein (P-gp), BCRP (breast cancer resistance protein), nucleoside transporters, hPEPT1 (human peptide transporter), OCTs (organic cation transporters), and ASBT (apical sodium-dependent bile acid transporter).

Active Transporter

The effectiveness and selectivity towards biological targets have always been the primary foci of drug development. However, phase II and III clinical trials of drug candidates often fail because of toxic effects and other unfavorable pharmacokinetic (PK) features including absorption, distribution, metabolism, and excretion (ADME). Early drug research now routinely includes in-vitro assessments of ADME characteristics to reduce attrition rates in later stages. Thanks to the explosion of computing power and the tremendous improvements in in silico modeling methods, high-throughput in vitro ADMET property screening tests have been established. Since active transporters are present on most barrier membranes and since their substrates and many medicines have similarities, they play an important role in ADMET modeling programs. Unfortunately, most prediction tools find it challenging to include the impacts of active transport because to our inadequate understanding of transporter mechanics. Despite this, a mountain of in vitro data has accumulated because to the growing fascination in these transporters. This led to the development of pharmacophore and QSAR models for a substantial number of these transporters. The complex role of transporters in drug disposition, including absorption, distribution, and excretion, may be better understood with the use of these transporter models. These are

1. **P-gp**

   An ATP-subordinate efflux carrier, P-glycoprotein (P-gp) transports a wide variety of substrates out of the cell. It improves renal and hepatic output while decreasing absorption, which in turn affects drug attitude. For example, it is well-known that P-gp restricts the gastrointestinal intake of paclitaxel, an anticancer medicine, and the central nervous system infiltration of HIV protease inhibitors. It is also responsible for the side effect of medication interactions during cancer treatment. Due to its significance in medication behavior and effective illness treatment, P-gp has attracted several efforts and is now the most extensively studied carrier, with abundant trial data.The BCRP

   One such ATP-dependent efflux transporter that imparts resistance to many anticancer drugs, including mitoxantrone and anthracyclines, is the breast cancer resistance protein (BCRP). The complex involvement of BCRP in drug disposition behavior is suggested by its expression in several organs and tissues, including the gut, liver, and brain, as well as its high levels of expression in haematological malignancies and solid tumors. Even while a candidate chemical may still be able to undergo BCRP transport if it does not meet the transport model, this does not mean it cannot. Since no model can include all conceivable chemical space, this limitation need to be taken into account by all predictive in silico models.

2. Nucleoside transporter

Natural nucleosides and their synthesized analogues, such as cladribine and zalcitabine, which are antiviral and anticancer medications, are transported via nucleoside transporters. distinct nucleoside transporters have distinct substrate specificities; for example, CNT1, CNT2, and CNT3 are concentrative transporters, whereas ENT1 and ENT2 are equilibrative transporters. When it comes to drug absorption, distribution, and excretion, the high-affinity, selective CNTs are mostly found in the epithelia of the gut, kidney, liver, and brain, in contrast to the ubiquitous broad-affinity, low-selective ENTs. Using pharmacophore and 3DQSAR modeling approaches, a more extensive analysis produced unique models for CNT1, CNT2, and ENT1. Two hydrophobic regions and a hydrogen bond acceptor on the pentose ring are shared characteristics of all models that are necessary for transport by nucleoside transporters.

3. hPEPT1

A wide variety of substrates are transported by the human peptide transporter (hPEPT1), an oligopeptide transport system with low affinity and high capacity. Drug absorption and excretion are impacted by its expression mostly in the intestines and kidneys. Three high-affinity substrates (Gly-Sar, bestatin, and enalapril) were used to construct a pharmacophore model. The model identified the hPEPT1 transport requirements as two hydrophobic features, one hydrogen bond donor, one hydrogen bond acceptor, and one negative ionizable feature.

4. ASBT

Intestinal epithelial cells and cholangiocytes exhibit the highly efficient and capacitive human apical sodium-dependent bile acid transporter (ASBT). It offers an extra intestinal target for better medication absorption by aiding the absorption of bile acids and their analogs. Based on the model, the transport requirements for ASBT are as follows: one hydrophobic center, one negative charge, one hydrogen bond donor, and one hydrogen bond acceptor.

5. **OCT**

   Many cationic medications are able to be taken up by the kidneys, liver, and gut epithelia via the organic cation transporters (OCTs). Organic cations (with a net positive charge at physiological pH) include a large number of pharmaceuticals and their byproducts. Three OCTs—OCT1, OCT2, and OCT3—have been cloned from various animals. The model proposes that human OCT1 has a single positive ionizable feature and three hydrophobic characteristics that are necessary for transport. There has been recent news about the molecular factors that determine substrate binding to rabbit OCT2 and human OCT2. The binding requirements of the two orthologs were identified and discriminated using 2D- and 3D-QSAR analysis.

6. **OATP**

   Many medications have an effect on plasma concentrations due to organic anion transporting polypeptides (OATPs), which actively transport these medicines across many different types of tissue membranes, including those in the brain, intestines, liver, and lungs. The wide substrate specificity of OATPs allows them to transport a wide variety of organic ions, including both anionic and cationic medicines.

7. **BBB- Choline Transporter**

   Although organic drug molecules may selectively pass across the blood-brain barrier (BBB), this makes medication administration to the brain problematic. The blood-brain barrier (BBB) vasculature expresses a number of transporters for nutrients and solutes, which might be used to deliver medications to the brain. We are particularly interested in organic cation transporters because of their potential use in delivering cationic chemicals to the central nervous system. Choline is a charged cation that may penetrate the blood-brain barrier and enter the central nervous system via a natural nutrition transporter called the BBB-choline transporter. Its structural needs may be better understood to aid in the prediction of BBB permeability, and its active transport helps choline-like molecules penetrate the BBB. Once better data from the cloned BBB-choline transporter is available, more precise in silico models might be created. Because charged cations do not diffuse easily across cell membranes in physiological settings, carrier-mediated transport is essential for choline absorption. There are now three groups of transporters that make up the choline transport system. Transport substrate, sodium dependency, tissue distribution, choline affinity, and susceptibility to the choline uptake inhibitor hemicholinium-3 (HC-3) are all unique characteristics of each transporter.

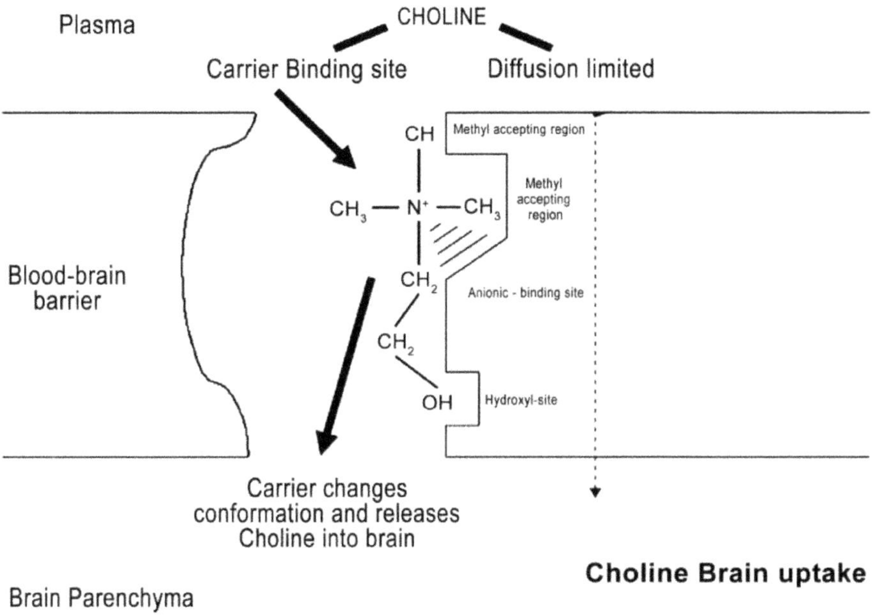

FIGURE 3 Depiction of choline blood-brain barrier permeation.

Table 1 Properties of Different Choline Transporters.

Protein Name	K_m for Choline	Sodium Dependency	Tissue Distribution	Substrates
CHT1	0.5-3 µm	Yes	Brain, Spinal Cord	Choline
CTL1	10-50 µm	No	Multiple tissues	Choline, Organic cation
CTL2	50-200 µm	Unknown	Placenta, lung	Choline
CTL3	Unknown	Unknown	Colon, Pancreas	Unknown
CTL4	Unknown	Unknown	Prostate, Colon	Thiamine Pyrophaste
CTL5	Unknown	Unknown	Multiple tissues	Unknown
OCT1	300-400 µm	No	Liver, Kidney	Organic cation
OCT2	100-500 µm	No	Kidney, Brain	Organic cation

CHT: High Affinity Choline Transporter, CTL: Choline Transporter like Protein, OTC: Organic cation Transporter,

Bibliography

1. Inazu, M. Choline transporter—like proteins CTLs/SLC44 family as a novel molecular target for cancer therapy. *Biopharm. Drug Dispos.* 2014, *35*, 431–449.

2. Kai Bittermann1, Kai-Uwe Goss. Predicting apparent passive permeability of Caco-2 and MDCK cell-monolayers: A mechanistic model. December 27, 2017.
3. Kim SH, Jackson AJ, Hunt CA. In silico, experimental, mechanistic model for extended-release felodipine disposition exhibiting complex absorption and a highly variable food interaction. PLoS One. 2014 Sep 30;9(9): e108392.
4. Loreto M. Valenzuela*, Andrea G. Reveco-Chilla, José M. del Valle. Modeling solubility in supercritical carbon dioxide using quantitative structure–property relationships. 6 July 2014.
5. Yulan Wang1, Jing Xing1, Yuan Xu1, Nannan Zhou, Jianlong Peng1, Zhaoping Xiong3, Xian Liu1, Xiaomin Luo1, Cheng Luo1, Kaixian Chen1, Mingyue Zheng1* and Hualiang Jiang1. In silico ADME/T modelling for rational drug design. Quarterly Reviews of Biophysics (2015), 48(4), pages 488–515.

UNIT III

Concept of Optimization, Optimization Parameters

When given a collection of options, optimization means picking the best one. "Simply said, optimization is the process of making anything more ideal, useful, or effective than it already is," says Merriam-Webster. "Optimize" means "make as perfect as feasible" in mathematical techniques. Optimal formulation is the goal of this technique. It denotes discovering the most efficient and effective way to do something, or making the most of something already in existence.

Choosing and processing components is what formulation development is all about. The goal of optimization is to learn the formulation's components and the processing parameters and ingredients that should be targeted. Quality selection is its primary function. Here is how optimization is defined in the context of pharmaceuticals: Optimization is the process of making the most of the available resources in an experiment by considering all of the variables that can affect the outcome. In the literature, optimization is used to describe any study of formulas. When developing projects, pharmacists often follow a systematic process of experimentation, making little adjustments to each variable until they reach a suitable conclusion. The pharmaceutical business currently use this optimization method.

Factorial Design

A factorial experiment is one in which there are two or more factors, each of which may take on a range of values. In 1926, Fisher invented the Factorial Design approach.

There are two types of factorial designs.

1. Full Factorial Design.
2. Fractional Factorial Design.

Full Factorial Design: Importantly, instead of changing each element independently, a complete factorial design changes all of the factors at once, making it feasible to test any conceivable combination of factors. The tester may look at both major impacts using this method.

As a condensed form of the complete factorial design, a fractional factorial design makes use of a subset of the available runs. Although there is a loss of information, a fractional factorial design makes better use of resources by decreasing the test's sample size.

The following are some of the most often used terms in factorial design:

Optimization: Finding the best way to employ the resources that are currently accessible while considering all the factors that impact decisions in each experiment is what it's all about. As ideal, efficient, or practical as may be achieved by picking the finest parts from a given range of possibilities. Thus, the optimal performance of an experiment is defined by the experimental settings used. In order to minimize formulation discrepancies, contemporary pharmaceutical optimization employs tests that are methodically designed.

Variables: Several elements have varying degrees of effect on the development of a product or process. Differences include quantitative and qualitative characteristics as well as independent and dependent ones. When it comes to independent factors, such as medication concentration or polymer composition, the investigator has complete control. The reaction of the final product (tablet/microsphere) to the effect of dependent factors, such as a medication release profile, is an example of a dependent variable. Any variable that may be expressed as a numerical value is considered quantitative. Example: concentration, pressure, and temperature. The kind of carrier or polymer is an example of a qualitative variable.

Factor: A factor is a predetermined variable, such concentration or temperature. Quantitative elements are numerically represented by values like 1%, 2%, and 3%; qualitative factors, on the other hand, are not numerical and include things like therapy, diet, labs, analyzers, batch of materials, and excipients.

Levels: A factor's levels are values or labels that have been ascribed to it.

Response: Calculated objective variables assess the connection between changes in the levels of each element and changes in response.

Effect: Is the link between different factors and their levels, as well as the change in reaction caused by changing the amount of a specific factor?

Screening Design

Experimental Design

Achieving a satisfactory dissolution rate with few trials is the fundamental concept for building an optimum pharmaceutical formulation in the creation of extended-release dosage forms. One of the most important things for pharmaceutical scientists is to conduct as few trials as possible when developing dosage forms; Design of Experiments (DoE) offers several benefits in this regard [1]. The factorial design necessitates 2k runs of experimentation to test k factors at 2 levels in this study. The number of runs increases proportionally with the number of factors or levels; for example, 4 factors at 2 levels require 16 runs to test, while 6 factors at 2 levels require 64 runs. The statistical method is useful because it may reduce the margin of error in variable determination when dealing with issues requiring a well-defined experimental design. In order to find the best formulation, researchers may use design of experiments (DOE) principles to examine different kinds of experimental designs, generate polynomial mathematical connections, and map the response [2-3]. Using a two-tiered Placket and Burman (PB) design, this experiment selects independent variables. Compared to the traditional methods of dosage form optimization and formulation, PB design has several advantages, including a shorter learning curve and more accurate results when choosing the optimal formulation. We have selected CS concentration, Eudragit concentration, MCC concentration, and Hardness as independent variables, together with their low and high levels, to investigate the cumulative percentage release of medication at 2, 4, 8, 14, and 20 hours, and to identify the burst impact by guaranteeing full drug release. According to reports, the most effective screening approach is the Placket and Burman design [4]. Developing a dosage form that is safe, effective, and user-friendly is the primary goal of quality by design (QbD).

The variables were correlated using the following polynomial equation with PB design.

$$Y = A0 + A1X1 + A2X2 + A3X3 + A4X4 + \ldots\ldots\ldots\ldots + AnXn$$

Where, Y is the response, A0 is the constant and A1 is the coefficients of the response [5]

Box-Behnken Experimental Design

Time and money are valuable resources, thus it's important to limit the number of runs without sacrificing the intended outcomes by picking the right mix of parameters. The complete factorial, also known as Box-Behnken, is often used for this purpose [6]. To reduce the time needed to produce pharmacological dosage forms, optimization using factorial design and analysis of the response surfaces are effective, methodical, and powerful approaches [7].

An appropriate one-way analysis of variance (ANOVA) was performed on the data acquired for the replies using linear, 2-FI, and quadratic models. In order to examine the impact of each independent variable on the dependent variables, the models were described and corresponding three-dimensional (3D) response surface plots and two-dimensional contour plots were generated using the Design Expert 8.0.7.1 program [8-10].

The nonlinear quadratic model equation produced by the BBD is of the form as below

R0+ b0 + b1X1 + b2X2 + b3X3 + b4X1X2 + b5X2X3 + b6X1X3 + b7X12 + b8X22 + b9X32

Where R0 = dependent variable or response;

X1, X2, and X3 = independent variable coded levels;

b0 = intercept; b1 to b9 = regression coefficients

Computers in Pharmaceutical Formulation

Pharmaceutical formulation, and especially the creation of novel drug delivery methods, has become an area where computers have become crucial tools. Microemulsions and pharmaceutical emulsions in particular have been the focus of much research due to their many potential uses as carriers for the enhancement of drug solubility, bioavailability, and targeted administration. In this paper, we'll look at how computers have helped pharmaceutical companies develop better emulsions and microemulsion drug carriers, and how such innovations have improved medication delivery while also benefiting the pharmaceutical sector. The development and optimization of drug formulations rely heavily on computational modeling. It provides helpful information on how drug molecules, excipients, and other components interact with one another, which helps researchers to anticipate how various formulations would behave in different environments. The physicochemical features of emulsions and microemulsions, which affect stability, droplet size, and drug release kinetics, may be better understood by computer simulations.

Development of Pharmaceutical Emulsions, Microemulsion Drug Carriers

Emulsions are biphasic systems composed of immiscible liquids, typically oil and water, stabilized by surfactants and co-surfactants. Computational tools aid in selecting the appropriate oil-water ratio, surfactant types, and concentration to achieve stable emulsions with desired properties. In addition, computational fluid dynamics (CFD) simulations help optimize the mixing process, ensuring uniform droplet size distribution, which is crucial for consistent drug delivery. By modeling the interactions between surfactants, oils, and water, researchers can predict emulsion stability, droplet coalescence, and Ostwald ripening, enabling the development of formulations with improved shelf life and bioavailability.

Microemulsions are thermodynamically stable systems composed of water, oil, surfactants, and co-surfactants, forming nanoscale droplets with enhanced Solubilization capacity. Computers aid in predicting the phase behavior and self-assembly of components to achieve microemulsion formulations with optimal drug-loading capabilities and controlled drug release profiles. Molecular dynamics simulations provide insights into the structure of microemulsion interfaces and interactions between components, contributing to the design of stable and efficient drug carriers. Moreover, virtual experiments using computational techniques help identify the most promising formulations before conducting laborious and resource-intensive experimental trials.

Computational tools have revolutionized pharmaceutical formulation, offering invaluable insights and predictive capabilities for the development of pharmaceutical emulsions and microemulsion drug carriers. By facilitating the design, optimization, and understanding of these innovative delivery systems, computers have paved the way for more efficient drug development processes, enhanced drug delivery, and improved patient outcomes. The synergy between computational modeling and experimental validation continues to shape the future of pharmaceutical formulation, ushering in a new era of precision and innovation in drug delivery systems.

Legal Protection of Innovative uses of Computers in R&D

Expertise in processing and ingredient selection is required for pharmaceutical formulation and development. The research and formulation of pharmaceutical products has seen a recent uptick in the usage of computer technologies. "Optimization" minimizes expenses while producing the ideal formulation. In pharmaceutical optimization, typically, a single variable is changed at a time in order to fix a problematic formulation. It is more intelligent to utilize computer tools (optimization technique) to find the right answer to a problem when the formulation is challenging.To optimize anything is to choose the best element or aspect out of a group of alternatives. Optimization refers to the steps taken to ensure that a design, system, or choice is as efficient and effective as possible. For optimization of a formulation, the formulator has two types of problems constrained problem and unconstrained problem. Constrained problems are those which have some physical restrictions placed on them where as unconstrained are independent. E.g. Formulator has to make a hardest tablet possible. This is unconstrained where as if it is being suggested that make hardest tablet which should disintegrate in less than 15 minutes. The restriction is placed and thus makes the problem more constrained type. There are a number of factors that go into the process of pharmaceutical formulation. There are two ways to classify them mathematically. Difference between independent and dependent variables. When a formulator makes a change to one or more independent variables, the dependent variables are the ones that follow suit as a result of that modification. A response's (the dependent variable) connection with the response surface's (the independent variable) is constant. The surface that is dependent on some variable.

New medications have a long way to go before they can be made accessible to the public due to the high costs and lengthy processes involved in pharmaceutical research and development. This book delves into the basics of computational fluid dynamics in pharmaceutical technology, computer-aided biopharmaceutical characterization, neural computing (including artificial neural networks, fuzzy logic, decision trees, evolutionary computing, genetic algorithms, and self-organizing maps), and chemometric methods with a focus on their use in process control. From initial concept to final product selection, all of these methods are vital for ensuring high-quality pharmaceutical goods and procedures. The book covers both the theory and practice of pharmaceutical technology, with plenty of examples of different ways in action. [11-14].

R&D is an ever-evolving process that has recently seen a shift toward the application of computer science in research and development. By leveraging computer science, teams are able to unlock new insights from data faster than ever before. From predictive analytics to artificial intelligence, these technologies have revolutionized how R&D teams can develop products more efficiently while staying ahead of their competitors.

Overview of Computer Science in Research and Development

Computer science is the study of algorithms and data structures that enable computers to solve problems. It involves creating algorithms that can be used by machines or programs to complete tasks efficiently and accurately. This includes developing software applications for specific purposes such as machine learning (ML), artificial intelligence (AI), natural language processing (NLP), image recognition, and robotics.

The application of computer science in research and development has become increasingly important due to its ability to help teams quickly analyze large amounts of data, automate processes, and uncover insights faster than ever before.

Benefits of Computer Science in R&D

The application of computer science in research and development provides numerous benefits.

1. Increased efficiency in analysis.
2. Improved accuracy.
3. Faster decision-making.
4. Better collaboration between team members.
5. Enhanced security measures.
6. Cost savings through automation.
7. Access to real-time insights into customer behavior patterns.
8. Improved customer experience through personalized services.
9. More accurate predictions based on historical trends and more reliable forecasting models.

Additionally, computer science helps organizations gain a competitive advantage by providing them with the ability to develop innovative products at a faster rate than their competitors while also reducing costs associated with product development cycles.

Challenges of Computer Science in R&D

While there are many advantages associated with the application of computer science in research and development, there are also some challenges that need to be taken into consideration. These include:

1. Ensuring compliance with regulations related to privacy or intellectual property rights.
2. Managing resources effectively.
3. Training personnel adequately so they can use the tools correctly.

4. Guarding against cyber threats.
5. Maintaining high levels of accuracy when dealing with large datasets.
6. Keeping up-to-date on new technologies being developed within the industry.

Benefits of Computer Science in R&D

Computer science has revolutionized the way research and development (R&D) teams work. With its powerful tools, computer science enables R&D teams to achieve greater efficiency and productivity in their projects.

1. **Increased Efficiency and Productivity**

   Computer science helps R&D teams become more efficient by automating mundane tasks such as data collection, analysis, and reporting. This allows them to focus on the creative aspects of their projects instead of spending time on tedious manual processes.

   Additionally, computer science provides access to a wide range of software that can be used to improve workflow management and project tracking which leads to increased productivity across the board.

2. **Improved Accuracy and Quality Control**

   Computer science also offers improved accuracy when it comes to data collection, analysis, and reporting due to its ability to quickly process large amounts of information with minimal errors or omissions. This makes it easier for R&D teams to identify potential problems before they arise which improves quality control throughout the entire product lifecycle from concept through commercialization stages.

3. **Reduced Costs and Time-to-Market**

   Finally, utilizing computer science in R&D projects reduces costs associated with labor-intensive activities like data entry or manual testing procedures. It also speeds up production times so products are able to reach the market faster.

There has been a sea change in the pharmaceutical R&D industry due to the introduction of cutting-edge computer technology. These advancements have transformed the way researchers analyze data, model molecules, and optimize drug candidates. The intersection of pharmaceutical R&D and computer science has introduced new challenges and opportunities, particularly in the realm of legal protection for innovative uses of computers. This essay deals into the legal aspects surrounding the protection of novel computer applications in pharmaceutical R&D, highlighting the importance of intellectual property rights and the potential challenges posed by patent law.

Intellectual Property Rights in Pharmaceutical R&D

When it comes to pharmaceutical research and development using computers, intellectual property (IP) rights such as patents, copyrights, and trade secrets are crucial for protecting the creative parts. In example, patents are very important because they let creators to have a monopoly on their innovations for a certain amount of time, preventing others from producing, using, or selling their ideas. In the context of pharmaceutical R&D, novel computer programs or algorithms used for drug discovery, molecular modeling, data analysis, and other innovative applications can be patented to protect the creators' rights and incentivize further research and innovation.

Challenges in Patenting Computer-Related Innovations

While the concept of patenting computer-related innovations in pharmaceutical R&D seems promising, certain challenges need to be addressed. One major challenge lies in defining the patent eligibility criteria for software-related inventions. Many countries have varying approaches to determine whether software innovations are eligible for patent protection. Striking a balance between encouraging innovation and avoiding the grant of overly broad patents that hinder future advancements is essential.

The Issue of Patentable Subject Matter

Patent law traditionally requires inventions to be tangible and fall under the categories of machines, processes, articles of manufacture, or compositions of matter. However, computer programs and algorithms are intangible and do not fit neatly into these categories. This poses a challenge in determining the patentability of software-related innovations in pharmaceutical R&D. To address this issue, some jurisdictions have introduced specific guidelines or tests to assess whether a software invention is eligible for patent protection, such as the "technical effect" or "technical solution to a technical problem" test.

Protecting Innovative Uses of Computers in Pharmaceutical R&D:

One way to address these challenges is by focusing on the practical application and technical aspects of computer-related innovations in pharmaceutical R&D. For instance, instead of claiming the software itself, innovators can seek patent protection for the specific processes, methods, or techniques that utilize the software to achieve a technical outcome. This approach aligns with the concept of solving a technical problem using the software, thus meeting the patent eligibility criteria in many jurisdictions.

So innovative uses of computers have revolutionized pharmaceutical R&D, enabling faster and more accurate drug discovery, optimization, and data analysis. Ensuring legal protection for these computer-related innovations is crucial for fostering continued progress in the pharmaceutical industry. While challenges exist, by carefully considering patent eligibility criteria and focusing on the technical aspects of the inventions, creators can successfully navigate the legal landscape and safeguard their innovative contributions. Ultimately, a balanced approach to intellectual property rights will encourage further exploration and development of cutting-edge technologies at the intersection of computer science and pharmaceutical research.

The Ethics of Computing in Pharmaceutical Research

There is no question that new ethical challenges have emerged with the introduction of computers, IT, and information systems. These challenges and conflicts have not only confronted practitioners grappling with novel predicaments but also engaged professional philosophers delving into the conceptual underpinnings of computer usage. These ethical issues extend beyond individual concerns stemming from practical experiences; they also encompass collective considerations entailing policy and procedural judgments. These overarching observations hold true not only in the broader context of computer utilization but also specifically in the realm of pharmaceutical research. Here, we want to investigate the difficulties and potential ethical implications of using computers in pharmacological research.

Ethical Issues: Privacy, Liability, Ownership, And Power

"Computer Ethics" by Deborah Johnson (3rd edition, 2001) is an excellent and succinct guide to exploring the field of computer ethics. This seminal book, which originally published as the first edition [15-16] and which is ranked #1 in the Philosopher's Index under "computer ethics," provides a theoretical framework that includes important topics including power, ownership, privacy, and responsibility. A large chunk of its analysis is still applicable and lasting, even though it emerged early in the short history of computer ethics.

Privacy

The concept of privacy has long been associated with what Justice Brandeis summed up more than a century ago as "the right to be allowed alone" [17]. To be more precise, it is the right of an individual to decide for themselves the kind, level, and means of disclosure of their personal information [18]. Essentially, this right bestows upon individuals the authority to govern the information shared about themselves, with the supplier typically retaining control over what is supplied [19]. The possibility of violating the right to privacy, in its widest or narrowest sense, becomes apparent within the framework of computer applications in pharmacological research.

Three major facets of the right to privacy have been defined by philosophers. For any intrusion that encroaches upon privacy, considerations of relevance, consent, and methodology come into play. Relevance entails the requirement for any intrusion into privacy to be directly pertinent to the matter under scrutiny. In the context of pharmaceutical research, a common concern may arise in the form of uncovering more about an individual than is pertinent to the research scope. In such cases, any extraneous information must be disregarded and promptly discarded.

The third facet addressing potential invasions of privacy stipulates that the approach used to inquire into an individual's private life should be routine and reasonable. In the realm of pharmaceutical research, researchers should abstain from contributing to the augmentation of available personal information. Moreover, given the advances in data mining techniques, it is incumbent upon researchers to adopt preventive measures and incorporate safeguards that prevent the identification of any individual subjects involved in the research.

In her work, Johnson extensively explores various facets related to liability, offering an essential distinction. Negligence, legal repercussions, the obligation of honesty, the nature of contracts, misrepresentation, and warranties (explicit and implicit) are all topics that fall under the umbrella of responsibility and computer usage [20]. When deciding whether software is a product or a service, a key difference emerges. In research settings, the distinction between software as a product and a service is more important than many of the other issues, which are less relevant to ethicists studying computer ethics.

The sale and utilization of software as a pre-packaged entity imbue it with the attributes of a product; thereby subjecting it to strict liability should defects arise. Yet, particularly in research scenarios, software is often custom-crafted for specific purposes, rendering it more akin to providing a service than a product. In instances where software serves distinct research objectives, exclusive liability may not rest solely upon the software provider. In such cases, clear and precise communication between the researcher and programmer becomes imperative. Elevating communication precision enhances the accuracy of research data, as underscored by Mason's observation [21-22] in the early stages of computer use that authenticity and correctness underpin accuracy.

In the pharmaceutical industry, a prevailing debate revolves around research visibility for potential drug users. Notably, certain companies, such as Eli Lilly and Company, pledge to make their research public, empowering individuals to assess drug efficacy independently. Scientific research inherently facilitates result sharing and replication among peers. This shift towards research visibility stands to diminish liability for drug manufacturers and researchers, bolster accuracy, and foster informed drug usage.

The pivotal matter of accuracy intertwines with liability considerations. As pharmacogenetics and personalized drug therapy trends gain momentum, the significance of accuracy and its ensuing liability escalates. However, this intensified emphasis on accuracy comes hand in hand with a deeper understanding of individuals. If the right to privacy demands safeguarding, stringent limitations on program accessibility, particularly in research-oriented programs, may be imperative. Thus, technological safeguards must be established to avert program intrusions, supplemented by stringent access controls dictated by well-defined policies and procedures. Individuals with strong ties to the program and its related institution bear the brunt of responsibility for program invasions and data breaches in the absence of adequate rules and clear processes.

Ownership

Among the intriguing philosophical inquiries related to computers, the status of software stands out as an enigmatic issue. Unlike conventional artistic forms such as paintings, music, or literature that exhibit similarities, computer software defies easy comparison. The legal domain has wrestled with this complexity, struggling to apply existing laws to software. Attempts to address software ownership have employed various strategies, all circumscribed by the right to property. However, given the unique nature of software, questions remain concerning its classification and protection.

The distinctiveness of software as property raises unresolved queries, adding to the discourse on its "uniqueness." The pharmaceutical research setting adds another layer of complexity to the strategies already used to protect ownership and property rights, such as copyrights, patents, encryption, trade secrets, confidentiality agreements, trustworthiness, and loyalty. The status of property in the realm of healthcare introduces another layer of complexity. Health is widely regarded by philosophers as inherently valuable, existing for its own sake. On the other hand, property ownership holds a subordinate place. Dilemmas emerge: Should property rights shield medical breakthroughs, even if publicizing medical knowledge could yield significant utilitarian gains? Framing this issue pits property rights against utility considerations. Alternatively, some scholars approach the conflict through the lens of competing justice concepts, such as Rawls' and Nozick's theories.

Consequently, ownership of exceptionally valuable medical knowledge, often embedded in software, may need to give way to utility or the right to healthcare. Although the ownership discourse seems intertwined with a profound conceptual puzzle, the practical reality highlights that programmers offering their expertise may possess ownership claims over research and its outcomes. Hence, effective communication between researchers and programmers not only enhances accuracy and addresses liability but also necessitates resolving property rights issues.

Power

According to Johnson, one of the most important issues in computer ethics is the distribution of power. In his analysis of computer ethics, Mason reinforced this view, stressing the need of accessibility. In light of Moor's claims, the issue of power has more significance. The computer revolution, according to Moor's theory, has gone through two stages: introduction and penetration. According to his theory, the current phase is the power stage, where computers' impact on various facets of human life, including politics, social dynamics, and legal systems, becomes paramount.

Amidst Moor's call for inquiry, divergent viewpoints have emerged. For instance, Joy contends that checks should be imposed on technology and its progression. Conversely, others, such as Weckert, express less pessimism and alarm regarding the implications of computer technology, particularly its effects on human existence. The ongoing debate surrounding computers and their societal implications underscores the need for attention in this domain. The intricate interplay of computers and social relations poses a complex query that extends beyond immediate resolution. This query engages broad issues encompassing property rights, distributive justice concepts, and the analysis of "power."

Examining "power" in a broad sense as capacity, Johnson dissects computer utilization across several themes. Topics covered include power dynamics (i.e., whether it is more concentrated or more diffuse), the role of computer experts in resolving these issues, the values embedded in computer programming, the effects on people with and without access to computers, the possibility of alienation as a result of computers, and how computer use may perpetuate the status quo. For researchers in pharmaceuticals utilizing computers, specific concerns center on whether computer use reinforces the existing status quo and the potential exclusion of certain groups or the incorporation of inherent biases. Yet, these concerns are inherently tied to broader inquiries involving justice comprehension and equitable resource distribution.

The complicated issues concerning the preservation of the status quo and the optimal distribution of power cannot be immediately addressed by analyzing the effects of computers' ubiquitous presence on the status quo or their contributions to power centralization or decentralization. In essence, C. P. Snow's call for increased interaction between scientists, humanists, and technologists remains relevant. Engaging in discussions, analyses, and discourse that incorporate the perspectives of all three disciplines can enrich the understanding of these multifaceted issues.

While our discussion does not offer an exhaustive analysis of computer usage in the pharmaceutical industry, as that falls within the realm of specialized philosophers conducting conceptual evaluations in computer ethics, we advocate for the involvement of applied philosophers in research teams. In the dynamic landscape of technology, applied philosophers, alongside technology experts, should contribute to crafting policy statements and codes of conduct

Top Ten major Ethical Violations in Scientific Research

1. Manipulating or distorting research data
2. Neglecting critical aspects of human-subject protocols
3. Concealing affiliations with companies benefiting from personal research
4. Engaging in relationships with students, research participants, or clients that could raise suspicions
5. Plagiarizing by using others' ideas without proper acknowledgment or consent
6. Illegitimate use of confidential information for personal research

7. Omitting contradictory data that challenge one's previous findings
8. Bypassing minor human-subject requirements
9. Overlooking the use of flawed data or questionable data interpretation by others
10. Altering study design, methodology, or outcomes under pressure from funding sources

11. Computers in Market Analysis

Computers have revolutionized various aspects of business operations, profoundly impacting both traditional and modern procedures. The scope, structure, and dynamics of the marketing industry have experienced significant changes due to the rise of computer technology. The evolving landscape of the market, coupled with the explosion of information, has led to the emergence of a new marketing paradigm. While traditional marketing has been perceived as an art by some and as science by others, the novel approach of "marketing engineering" has gained traction. This term encapsulates the utilization of computer-based methodologies to analyze and develop marketing strategies that align with contemporary market trends [23-30].

A comprehensive market analysis, centred on specific industries, leverages the power of computers to delve into market dynamics and trends. Segmentation, a critical process in market research, seeks to understand distinct market segments. To define a "relevant market," in-depth research into market structures and processes is essential. The identified relevant market serves as a pivotal focus for companies' activities. Proper classification and division of markets facilitate the identification of related markets. In this context, a computer-based information system refers to a system that collects, processes, and communicates data directly to support strategic marketing decisions. This encompasses a wide range of resources, including but not limited to databases, spreadsheets, MIS, fuzzy logic, A.N.N.s, marketing and executive databases, decision support systems, and more.

There are various benefits of using computer technology into marketing:

12. Enhanced Marketing Precision

Computers empower marketers to analyze and manage vast consumer data, demographics, shopping history, and preferences. This knowledge enables personalized and targeted campaigns with greater precision, connecting products with specific customer groups.

13. **Increased Campaign Capacity**

    Cloud computing allows marketers to scale up computing capacity as needed, ensuring optimal performance during demand peaks. This is particularly valuable for handling large-scale campaign responses and test marketing.

14. **Automation of Marketing Campaigns**

    Marketing automation streamlines processes by analyzing customer responses and tailoring subsequent interactions based on their level of interest. This results in more effective follow-up communications and sales calls.

15. **Efficient Sales Support**

    Computer technology enables the digital distribution of marketing materials, providing authorized users with access to content such as brochures, presentations, and product data sheets. This controlled access enhances content distribution and usage.

16. **Improved Collaboration**

    Desktop videos and web-conferencing tools facilitate collaboration among sales, product development, and marketing teams. Teams can swiftly communicate, review proposals, and make decisions without the need for physical meetings.

17. **Web-Based Promotion**

    The internet offers a global advertising channel, encompassing in-text ads, banners, emails, and video ads. Online advertising can be cost-effective compared to traditional mediums, making it attractive to start-ups.

18. **Market Research**

    Computers enable efficient market research by utilizing surveys, data collection, and competitor analysis. Online survey tools simplify data collection and customer feedback, enhancing research capabilities.

19. **Creating Advertisements for Other Media**

    Computer technology aids in designing layouts for print media and editing videos for audio and TV commercials. Graphic designers and media experts utilize computers to enhance the quality of multimedia advertising.

20. **Distribution**

    Digital distribution through computers allows companies to reach customers remotely, eliminating the need for physical storefronts.

This is particularly advantageous for small businesses seeking nationwide reach without significant start-up costs.

So the integration of computer technology has reshaped the marketing landscape, offering numerous benefits such as precision, automation, collaboration, and cost-effective promotion. Embracing these technological advancements empowers businesses to effectively navigate the ever-changing market and maintain a competitive edge.

Bibliography

1. Alonso MJ, Cran LP, Lorenzo-Lamosa ML, Vila-Jato JL. Development of new chitosan–cellulose multicore micro-particles for controlled drug delivery. European Journal of Pharmaceutics and Biopharmaceutics. 1998; 45(1): 49-56.
2. Boca Raton, FL: CRC Press, Taylor & Francis Group. Balfagón, A.C., Serrano Hernanz, A., Teixido, J, and Tejedor-Estrada, R.(2010) 'Comparative study of neural networks and least mean square algorithm applied to the optimization of cosmetic formulations', Int. J.Cosmet. Sci, 32: 376-86.
3. Brandeis LD, Warren SD. The right to privacy. Harvard Law Rev 1890;4,5:193–220.
4. Cochran, W.G.; Cox, G.M. *Experimental designs,* 2nd ed; Wiley: New York, **1992**, pp. 335-339.
5. Couper MP, Traugott M, Lamias M. Web survey design and administration. Public Opinion Quarterly. 2001; 65:230–253.
6. Dayal, P., Pillay, V., Babu, R.J., Singh, M., 2005. Box–Behnken experimental design in the development of a nasal drug delivery system of model drug hydroxyurea: characterization of viscosity, in vitro drug release, droplet size and dynamic surface tension. AAPS Pharm Sci Tech, 6: E573–E585.
7. Dillman, D. A. (2007), Mail and Internet surveys: the tailored design method — 2007 update with new internet, visual, and mixed-mode guide, Wiley, Hoboken, NJ.
8. Freid C. An anatomy of values: problems of personal and social choice. Cambridge: Harvard University Press, 1970.
9. Hamed, E., Sakr, A., 2001. Application of multiple response optimization technique to extended release formulations design. J. Control. Release, 73: 329–338.
10. Imperial COE 2006. Qualitative and quantitative research. Referred 25.11.2013 http://www.icoe.org/webfm_send/1936.

11. Johnson DG. Computer ethics, third edition. Englewood Cliff, N.J.: Prentice Hall, 2001.
12. Kumar, K.J., Panpalia, G.M., and Priyadarshini, S. (2011) 'Application of artificial neural networks in optimizing the fatty alcohol concentration in the formulation of an o/w emulsion', Acta Pharm, 61: 249-56.
13. Kumari, K.P.; Shankar, G.G.; Prabhakar, T. Optimisation of L-asparaginase production by Streptomyces griseoluteus WS3/1 using experimental methods. *J. Pharm. Biomed. Sci.,* **2011**, *10*(11), 1-6.
14. Li S., Kinman R., Duan Y., and Edwards J. S. Computer-Based Support for marketing strategy development. European journal of marketing, 2000; 34(5/6): 551-575.
15. Li S., Kinman R., Duan Y., and Edwards J. S. Computer-Based Support for marketing strategy development. European journal of marketing, 2000; 34(5/6): 551-575.
16. Malah YEI, Nazzal S. Hydrophilic matrices: Application of Placket–Burman screening design to model the effect of POLYOX–carbopol blends on drug release. International Journal of Pharmaceutics. 2006; 309(1): 163-70.
17. Mason RO. Four ethical issues of the information age. MIS Quarterly 1986; 10 (March):4–12.
18. Moulai Mostefa, N., Hadj Sadok, A., Sabri, N., and Hadji, A. (2006) 'Determination of optimal cream formulation from long-term stabilityinvestigation using a surface response modelling', Int. JCosmet. Sci, 28: 211-18.
19. Prince J. Negligence: Liability for defective software. Oklahoma Law Rev 1980;33:848–55.
20. Prusty A, Gupta BK, Mishra AK. The Application of the Box-Behnken Design Response Surface Methodology to Study Optimized Formulation Variables on the Drug Release Pattern of Benidipine Hydrochloride. Drug Delivery Letters 2022; 12(1): 62-73.
21. Rahali, Y., Pensé-Lhéritier, A.M., Mielcarek, C., and Bensouda, Y. (2009) 'Optimization ofcream formulation from long-term stabilityinvestigation using a surface response modelling', Int. J.Cosmet. Sci, 28: 211-18.
22. Rath, S.; Gupta, B.K.; Bala, N.N.; Dhal, H.C. Formulation and optimization of immediate release telmisartan tablets using full factorial design. *Int. J. Appl. Pharm.,* **2011**, *3*(3), 587-610.

23. Schwartz, J.B.; O'Connor, R.E.; Schnaare, R.L. *Modern pharmaceutics: Optimization techniques in pharmaceutical formulation and processing,* 4th ed; Banker, G.S.; Rhodes, C.T., Eds.; Marcel Dekker, Inc.: New York, USA, **2002**, pp. 607-626.
24. Shih, T.-H. and Fan, X. , 'Response rates and mode preferences in web-mail mixedmode Surveys: a meta-analysis', International Journal of Internet Science 2007; 2, 59.
25. Silvius, G. Does ROI Matter Insights into the True Business Value of IT. The Electronic Journal Information Systems Evaluation, 2006; 9**,** 93-104.
26. Singh, B., Chakkal, S.K., Ahuja, N., 2006. Formulation and optimization of controlled release muco adhesive tablets of atenolol using response surface methodology. AAPS Pharm Sci Tech, 7: E1–E9.
27. Tourangeau R, Smith TW. Asking sensitive questions: the impact of data collection mode, question format and question context. Public Opin Q 1996; 60:275–304.
28. Vehovar, V. and Manfreda, K. L. (2008), 'Overview: online surveys', in Fielding, N. G., Lee, R. M. and Blank, G. (eds), The SAGE handbook of online research methods, SAGE Publications Ltd, London.
29. Velasquez MG. Business ethics—concepts and cases, 5th ed. Upper Saddle River, NJ: Prentice Hall. 2002.
30. Wright RA. Information as a commodity. In: Bynum TW, Maner W, John L. Fisher JL, editors, Computing and privacy. New Haven: Southern Connecticut State University Press, 1992;20–30.

UNIT IV

Computer Aided Biopharmaceutical Characterization

Gastrointestinal Simulation

The goal of this study is to develop and evaluate in silico methods that can predict drug absorption using the data set(s) of input elements that have been chosen, and that can identify crucial factors (such as drug physicochemical qualities and dosage form factors) that influence drug in vivo performance. Numerous factors, including the physicochemical qualities of the medication, physiological variables, and formulation-related factors, influence the absorption of the drug in the body. There has been a lot of difficulty in using in silico models to predict pharmacokinetics characteristics.

Classification of Models: The physiology of the gastrointestinal system as it pertains to drug transit, solubility, and absorption has been the focus of intensive efforts to create and disseminate dynamic models.

Types of Models

Different types of model are

1. Advanced dissolution, absorption and metabolism (ADAM) model
2. Grass model
3. GI-transit-absorption (GITA) model
4. Compartmental Absorption and Transit (CAT) model
5. Advanced CAT (ACAT) model
6. Integrated in commercial software packages, such as Gastroplus™, SimCYP, PK-sim ®
7. Dynamic Models: When coupled with pharmacokinetic (PK) models, dynamic models may assess plasma concentration-time profiles and forecast both the proportion of dosage absorbed and the rate of drug absorption. Compared to in vivo research, this

model has the ability to test virtual substances with less investment of time and money. This results in a significant decrease in the amount of tests, as well as the time and money needed for compound creation and selection.

Aid Justification of Biowaivers: It evaluates the correlation between in vitro and in vivo data that estimates the impact of medicine and/or formulation qualities on the absorption profile that results from food and predicts the effects of food. Studies using GI Simulation technology (GIST) are conducted to forecast the absorption of oral drugs.

Predicting the pharmacokinetic and pharmacodynamic effects of medications in people and certain animals is the primary function of GastroPlusTM, which are state-of-the-art computer systems. The ACAT model, which is an upgraded version of the original CAT device, is known as GastroPlusTM. This model of semi-physiological absorption takes into account both current understanding of gastrointestinal (GI) physiology and the idea of the Biopharmaceutics Classification System (BCS). Also, the ACAT model of the human gastrointestinal system is made up of nine interconnected sections, or compartments, that stand in for various parts of the tract: the stomach, duodenum, two sections of the jejunum, three sections of the ileum, caecum, and ascending colon. The unreleased, unreported, dissolved, and absorbed drug are further separated into these compartments. Several differential equations characterize the drug's movement between the various sub-compartments.

Model Construction

It all begins with gathering data for modeling and simulation. Several input parameters are needed by mechanistic absorption models; these values may be found empirically or calculated in silico. All four BCS medication classes were included in the reported research, along with various dose forms such as solutions, suspensions, immediate and controlled release (CR) formulations, and more. We simulated either fasting or fed human or animal physiologies, depending on the study's goals. We have also investigated the possibility of using the Single Simulation or Virtual Trial modes, which allow us to include inter-subject variability into the model.

GI Simulation: General modeling and Simulation strategy

To demonstrate the basic procedures of utilizing GastroPlusTM for mechanistic modeling and simulation to forecast oral medication absorption, Gliclazide (GLK) was used as the model drug. Within the gastrointestinal (GI) pH range, the solubility of GLK, an ampholyte, varies with pH. The BCS has determined that GLK satisfies the requirements for a medication with poor solubility. The in vivo experiments reveal that GLK is almost entirely absorbed after oral treatment, although at a sluggish and unpredictable pace.

Parameter Sensitivity Analysis

It is of the utmost importance to comprehend the impact of different formulation factors and drug physicochemical qualities on anticipated PK profiles. The GastroPlusTM Parameter Sensitivity Analysis (PSA) tool makes this kind of assessment possible. Parametric sampling and analysis (PSA) is keeping all parameters at their baseline values while methodically adjusting one parameter at a time within a set range using previous information. Alternatively, a three-dimensional PSA can be conducted, varying two parameters simultaneously to assess their combined impact. Additionally, PSA can aid in constructing an optimized design space based on selected parameters. Use this tool when you need to estimate the values of physicochemical properties or when your model predictions don't match up with in vivo data. When this occurs, analysts may use PSA to fine-tune input parameters and develop an absorption model that is unique to each medication.

Predicting the impact of inter-individual variability in PK characteristics on medication absorption is another important use of PSA in relation to highly variable medicines. You may save time, effort, and resources during the pre-formulation procedures by using this predictive capacity as a guidance in formulation design. To determine the expected rate and amount of GLK absorption, PSA was used to evaluate the impact of certain formulation factors (effective particle radius, drug particle density) and drug physicochemical qualities (solubility, permeability). With the exception of human effective permeability, which varied between half a value and two times the input value, all of the other parameters were systematically altered from a tenth to a one-tenth of the actual input sizes. According to PSA results, the percentage of GLK absorbed (Fa) was only little impacted by changes in drug particle density and effective particle radius. The effect on bioavailability (Fa > 85%) of a tenfold decrease in solubility was insignificant. But GLK absorption rates were lower when particles were either bigger, denser, or had lower solubility values than what was employed in the simulations. Crucially, the absorption profile of the medicine was unaffected by changes in input effective permeability.

Parameter sensitivity analysis, in conclusion, is a vital resource for pharmacokinetics researchers seeking to comprehend the impact of formulation factors and drug characteristics on PK profiles. This method provides insights into optimizing drug-specific absorption models, supporting formulation design decisions, and predicting the impact of inter-individual variability on drug absorption.

Drug absorption profiles were unaffected by changes in input effective permeability, according to the data. An analysis of parameter sensitivity shows how various input parameters affect drug absorption percentage (a), maximum clearance (C max) (b), and time to maximum concentration (t max) (c). The values used in the simulations for each parameter are shown at the center of the x-axis, and a dotted line on the horizontal represents complete absorption (>85% drug absorbed).

Virtual Trial For formulations still in the works, it's crucial to account for potential inter-subject variability in oral medication bioavailability. With GastroPlusTM's Virtual Trial function, it is possible to virtually test the impact of population variability and/or the combined effect of formulation factors with imprecise values. Stochastic simulations, whereby the values of the chosen variables are drawn at random from predefined distributions (specified as means with coefficients of variation (CV%) in absolute or log space), may be run on a variety of virtual topics using this capability. It is common practice to estimate CV% values by consulting existing literature or drawing on prior information. The simulation results are shown as means and coefficients of variation for the following parameters: % of medication absorbed, bioavailability, t max, C max, and AUC values. Additionally, the bottom and top values for each of these parameters attained throughout the trials are also included. In order to run the simulation, we employed a set of randomly chosen stochastic variables with predefined coefficients of variation in log normal space, all falling within the range of the means. Twelve subjects were used in the virtual trials, which is the same number as in the clinical study. The results were shown as a mean Cp vs. time profile with 90% confidence intervals around the mean. Additionally, Cp vs. time curves for 25, 75, and 100% probability of simulated patient data were generated. All of the observed clinical data fell within the minimal and maximal individual patient simulations, according to the simulation results. This indicates that the variability in the observed clinical results is a product of the CV% values used for the log normal distributions of the stochastic variables. It followed that the variability in the clinical data might be predicted using virtual trial simulations based on the assumed distribution of the chosen variables.

FED VS Fasted State Many processes, including changes to gastrointestinal tract physiology, drug solubility and dissolution, and drug penetration, may be at work while food is present, all of which might influence medication absorption. As an example, lipophilic medications are known to exhibit enhanced solubilization in the presence of meals, which is caused by larger concentrations of bile salt and lipids. This leads to increased systemic exposure of the drug. Predicting drug absorption in animals using in silico modeling involves taking into account drug-specific characteristics like permeability, biorelevant solubility, ionization constant(s), dose, metabolism, distribution data, etc., in addition to prior knowledge of gastrointestinal physiology in both the fasted and fed states. For the fasting and fed states, biorelevant solubility was assessed in a variety of media, including simulated human stomach fluid, simulated human intestinal fluid, and upper and lower colonic fluid. By manipulating physiological variables and loading the proper solubility data into the three ACAT compartments (stomach, intestine, and colon), we were able to mimic the impact of food. To determine each drug's dietary impact, we compared the area under the curve (AUC) or C max between the fasting, fed, and high-fat situations. To test how well the simulations worked, we compared the predicted and actual plasma concentration-time profiles and dietary effects over a range of dosages. Findings showed that for all six chemicals, GI modeling using GastroPlusTM accurately predicted plasma exposure in fasting, fed, and high-fat settings.

In Vitro Dissolution and *In Vitro–In Vivo* Correlation

The United States Food and Drug Administration (FDA) defines an in vitro in vivo correlation (IVIVC) as a mathematical model that predicts the link between an oral dosage form's *in vitro* characteristic and relevant in vivo response. The quantity or rate of drug absorption or plasma concentration is the in vivo response, while the in vitro attribute is the rate or extent of drug dissolution or release (FDA, 1997). Improving our knowledge of how drugs work in both laboratory and living organism settings is a primary goal of pharmaceutical product development. A drug's in vivo performance may be anticipated from its in vitro behavior by the effective creation and use of an IVIVC. In addition to easing regulatory burdens, improving product quality, and serving as a substitute for bioequivalence investigations, a relevant IVIVC may be established. The importance of IVIVC in pharmaceutical product development has grown since the groundbreaking studies by Nelson (1957) and Edwards (1951) that linked the in vivo appearances of theophylline and aspirin after oral administration with their dissolution rates. Specifically, while developing IVIVC models, it is important to keep in mind the novel lipophilic drug candidates that have limited water solubility.

The process of logically associating a dosage form's physico-chemical properties or characteristics with its biological properties or parameters developed from those properties. What the FDA (Food and Drug Administration) describes An in vitro attribute of a dose form and its corresponding in vivo response may be described using a predictive mathematical model called IVIVC. Dissolving or release rates are examples of in vitro properties, while plasma drug concentrations and absorption rates are examples of in vivo responses.

Since the rate-limiting step in the appearance of the drug into the systemic circulation is the dissolution or release of the drug from the formulation, it is possible to establish a relationship between the release of the drug in vitro and its release in vivo or absorption into the systemic circulation for controlled-release or extended-release formulations. If this relationship holds, then the in vitro solubility of a medication may be used to forecast its plasma concentration time profile. Two or more formulations with distinct release characteristics are often used to build such a connection. Establishing a connection using three or more formulations is highly suggested. But if the drug's solubility is unaffected by the dissolving parameters (such as pH, apparatus agitation rate, etc.), then this kind of association may be shown with only one formulation. Setting up a predictive IVIVC has multiple benefits: first, it helps you understand the drug product's release properties better; second, it reduces the number of in vivo studies required to approve and keep a drug product on the market, which is good for the economy and easier on regulators. Using the anticipated plasma concentration time profile, it is also possible to establish clinically relevant dissolving requirements.

If the correlation can accurately predict the C max and AUC within 20%, then it is considered a significant and predictive IVIVC (FDA advice for industry, 1997b). To determine how predictable the correlation is, you may use one of two methods: (1) The capacity to anticipate the pharmacokinetic profile of the formulations used to establish the correlation is known as internal predictability. (2) The capacity to discern the profile of a lot or formulation that was not utilized to establish the IVIVC is known as external predictability. According to the US IVIVC advice for industry and the EMA's August 2012 guidelines, a bioequivalence study may be skipped in the US and EU if the reference and test are expected to have the same C max and mean AUC within a 20% margin of error.

Categories of *In Vitro–In Vivo* Correlations

Level A Correlation

At its most basic level, level A correlation is a one-to-one correspondence between the rate of drug absorption from a dosage form in vivo and its rate of solubility in vitro. The percentages of medication release and absorption are compared in a level A correlation. The Wagner-Nelson or Loo-Riegelman methods, as well as direct mathematical deconvolution, which involves mathematically separating the blood level into an absorption component and a disposition component, are common ways to determine the proportion of medicine that is absorbed. The development of a point-to-point correlation is the primary benefit of a Level A correlation. Efficacy data from in vivo plasma concentration-time profiles and dissolution data from in vitro experiments are used. An in vitro solution profile may stand in for in vivo performance when a Level A correlation is shown. Further human studies are not required to justify changes to the production location, mode of manufacture, raw material supply, small formulation modifications, or even product strength when employing the same formulation. If the in vitro dissolution test has a level A correlation, it may be used as a clinically relevant quality control tool to predict how well a drug product would work in vivo.

Level B Correlation

The statistical moment concept is used in level B correlation, which compares the mean in vitro dissolution time to either the mean residence time (MRT)2 or the mean in vivo dissolution time (MDT). The in vivo and in vitro data are both used in level B correlation, which is not a point-to-point correlation. Parameter values may be the same across profiles. On its own, the Level B connection is insufficient to warrant changes to the formulation, the manufacturing location, the supplier of excipients, the quality from batch to batch, etc.

Level C Correlation

There is no point-to-point relationship in a Level C connection. A Level C correlation is used when there is only one point of connection between two pharmacokinetic parameters, like AUC and Cmax, and a dissolution parameter, such percent dissolved at a certain time. Although it has limited use, level C correlation is helpful for formulation selection and development. The quantity of medication dissolved at different time points in the dissolution profile is related to one or more pharmacokinetic parameters of interest using multiple level C correlations. Generally speaking, developing a Level A correlation may be within reach if one can establish many Level C correlations. The following are a few instances of Level C correlation.

Dissolution rate versus absorption rate. A quicker dissolving rate could lead to a quicker appearance of the medicine in the plasma if the drug's dissolution is the rate limiting factor. There could be a link between how quickly a medicine dissolves and how quickly the body absorbs it. Finding the absorption rate is sometimes trickier than finding the peak absorption time. As a result, absorption time may be used to establish a connection between dissolution and absorption data. In the study of in vitro-in vivo drug correlation, the absorption time for the preparation may be used to differentiate between drugs with slow absorption and those with quick dissolution. A consistent dose of medication needs a certain length of time to be absorbed, and this is called the absorption time. There was a linear relationship between the preparations' dissolving times and their absorption times in a research using three sustained-release aspirin formulations (Levy et al., 1965). Absorption of aspirin was shown to be highly reliant on the rate of dissolution, according to the findings of this investigation.

For regulatory reasons, level D correlation—which includes rank order and qualitative analysis—is not appropriate. there helps in processing or formulating procedures, although there isn't a formal connection.

Methodology for Establishing Correlation

Developing the medicinal product with different release rates—slow, medium, quick, or even just one rate when dissolution is independent—enables the development of the correlation. In vivo concentration investigations of plasma bioavailability (BA) are carried out employing methodologies such as Wagnernelson. The time required for 50% absorption divided by the time required for 50% dissolution is the formula for the intensity factor. In order to determine the correlation, take the in vivo time (T) and divide it by the intensity factor to get the matching in vitro time point. The formation of correlations is influenced by factors including stereochemistry and the first-pass effect.

Percent of drug dissolved versus percent of drug absorbed. A linear connection may be found by comparing the percentage of drug absorbed to the percentage of drug dissolved if a drug is absorbed entirely after dissolution. To get an approximation of in vivo dissolution, one must choose an adequate dissolution media and swirl the mixture slowly while dissolving.

The quantity and rate of drug absorption throughout the time of observation may fluctuate due to a little change in formulation, as aspirin is absorbed quickly. A change in the product's dissolving rate could go unnoticed if the medicine is absorbed slowly, as happens when absorption is the rate-limiting phase. Here, the absorption rate of the medicine would be very poor, regardless of the rate of dissolution.

Evaluation of Predictability

To prove that a medicinal product's in vivo performance prediction is reliable across different in vitro dissolution release rates and manufacturing variations, an In Vitro-In Vivo Correlation (IVIVC) evaluation is required.

Biowaiver Considerations

Biowaivers refers to the situations in which *in vivo* BE studies can be substituted with the relevant *in vitro* data.

Bioequivalence studies for generic pharmaceutical drugs may be waived via a regulatory process known as a biowaiver. To prove that the generic version of a medicine has the same bioavailability (the amount and rate of drug absorption into the circulation) as the original drug, bioequivalence tests are necessary.

There are two main considerations for biowaiver:

1. The drug substance(s) in the test and reference products must be identical.
2. The test and reference products must belong to the same Biopharmaceutics Classification System (BCS) class.

Drugs are categorized into four groups according to the BCS, which takes into account their solubility and permeability. Class I medicines are the most bioavailable because of their high solubility and permeability. Due to their poor permeability and high solubility, Class II medicines may need biowaiver investigations in cases where the reference and test products have different formulations. Class III medicines are often subject to biowaiver investigations because to their high permeability and poor solubility. Class IV drugs have low solubility and low permeability, and are not eligible for biowaiver. In addition to the BCS class, other factors that may be considered for biowaiver include the drug's molecular weight, the presence of excipients, and the route of administration. The biowaiver procedure can be a significant time and cost savings for generic drug developers. However, it is important to note that not all drug products are eligible for biowaiver. If you are considering a biowaiver for your product, you should consult with a regulatory expert to ensure that you meet all of the requirements.

Regulatory bodies often use one of two biowaiver schemes: the BCS-based system, which calls for the test and reference products to have fast or very rapid dissolving profiles in pH 1.2, 4.5, or 6.8 media, or the IVIVC method. The FDA has limited the IVIVC-based approach to XR product applications, and biowaivers for IR drug products can only be requested for substances that are highly soluble and permeable (BCS class I), when the drug product dissolves (very) quickly and has a similar dissolution profile to the reference product. Some medications in BCS class II and III are now eligible for biowaivers if their high permeability is at 85% absorbed and their dose-to-solubility ratio at pH 6.8 is 250 mL or less, according to recommendations released by the EMA and the WHO. This is because these pharmaceuticals dissolve extremely quickly. It was also mentioned that the biowaivers idea should be further eased for BCS II and III medications. For example, BCS class II pharmaceuticals may be biowaived if they dissolve fully throughout the GI passage, and BCS class III compounds can be biowaived if they dissolve swiftly.

Computer Simulation in Pharmacokinetics and Pharmacodynamics

To simulate something is to imitate it, and algorithms allow computers to do just that. In this topic mimic the pharmacokinetic and pharmacodynamic to know about how the drug will react with the body and also how the body will react with the drug respectively. There is mainly 4 level of the simulation of pharmacokinetics and pharmacodynamic.

The modern age has been ushered in by technological advancements, and technology-driven discovery has become an integral part of increasing R&D productivity and designing novel chemical entities, such as drug candidates, for use against a wide range of biological targets. Pharmacokinetic characteristics, often referred to as ADME (absorption, distribution, metabolism, and excretion), have lately been associated with drug candidate failures in the latter stages of drug discovery and development. ADME models and AI-driven computer simulations, of differing degrees of sophistication, have been created to solve this problem and aid in the screening of enormous datasets of chemicals. These models have produced tools that are more efficient than conventional methods in terms of speed, simplicity, and cost. Drug pharmacokinetics and pharmacodynamic are studied with the use of computer simulation. A drug's pharmacokinetics (PK) refers to how it moves through your system and how it's used, while its pharmacodynamic (PD) examines how your body responds to the medicine [49-54]. Drug development and clinical practice in pharmacology rely on pharmacokinetics (PK) and pharmacodynamics (PD). The effectiveness and safety of drugs are heavily dependent on the cooperation of these two fields. In order to better understand and optimize medication behavior, researchers and doctors have come to rely on computer simulation. This technology allows them to make educated judgments and create treatment regimens that are successful. So we may say AI based Computer simulations are used to optimize drug dosing for individual patients, taking into account factors such as age, weight, and renal function. This personalized approach improves drug efficacy and minimizes the risk of adverse effects. Simulation can predict drug concentration-time profiles based on patient data, facilitating therapeutic drug monitoring. By adjusting doses according to the predicted response, clinicians can maintain drug levels within the therapeutic window. Generally there are mainly 4 level of the simulations of pharmacokinetics and pharmacodynamic.

Computer simulations of the complete organism at Level 1 employ two methods: the PK/PD model and the PBPK model. Two approaches to modeling a drug's effects on an organism as a whole are the PK/PD model and the PBPK model. Using the PK/PD paradigm, which stands for pharmacokinetic and pharmacodynamic, the exposure-response link is represented. When combined with a sick state model, this model may be described using a linear, E max, or Sigmoid E max model. In order to create a PK/PD research methodology, this model is used to collect data on pharmacokinetics in vitro and in vivo. Along the path from exposure to response, pharmacodynamics and pharmacokinetics operate as markers. A physiology-based pharmacokinetic (PBPK) model incorporates the effects of blood and lymph flow into a multi-compartmental model to predict the ADME of a synthetic or natural chemical substance in a person. Many physiological organs of the body are represented in this model by separate compartments connected by the circulatory blood stream.

Similarly in Level 2 Computer simulations of isolated tissue and organ, Heart, kidney, brain; liver can be a subject of mathematical modelling research which can be carried out with distributed blood tissue model that is known as BTEX model. This is the first ever research on the biodegradation of BTEX (Benzene, Toluene, and Xylene isomer). Benzene, Toluene, and an ortho, meta, or para Xylene derivative make up the new BTEX model. The competitive inhibition, toxicity, and creation of the hazardous intermediate underlie this synergistic and/or antagonistic interaction during biodegradation of the BTEX molecule.

The third level is simulation of cell, which is mainly used in biomedical research. Using an online respiratory model, researchers have created a computer simulation of a full cell and made it accessible to their user network. The Cell ML website also provides an online respiratory of the biophysical model. The directed network may be easily implemented on a computer, making it a straightforward method for modelling the intricate interaction between cells or even inside the intracellular milieu.

Finally the level 4 include simulation of protein and genes and the goal of this method was to use an ordinary differential equation to map genetic information onto a network, with the hope of identifying the gene(s) responsible for a disease's susceptibility. Clinical data provided significant insight into the underlying disease process, allowing researchers to use simulation to pharmacology in the area of HIV/AIDS treatment creating a novel gene sequence may aid in the protein identification, translation, and transcription.

Computers in Clinical Development

Thanks to recent advancements in computer hardware and software, it is now feasible to conduct clinical trials on novel drug molecules in a rapid, efficient, and trustworthy way. Therefore, the design, development, and selection of hardware and software for these systems must be carefully considered. In order to carry out effective clinical trials, it is essential to have thorough and trustworthy systems for collecting and managing data..

Clinical Data Collection and Management

Managing clinical trial data encompasses a series of procedures that need to be effectively carried out to produce accurate clinical, regulatory, and administrative data to a centralized destination, such as a coordinating center, data hub, or resource center. While these practices in still greater trust in the outcomes of clinical trials, the evolution of technology has brought about new obstacles that require attention. Among these challenges are expenses, the learning curve, changes in responsibilities, and handling unexpected occurrences. The time it takes to get from the last patient appointment to the final database lock out is cut in half. Reduce query rates and eliminate duplicate data input by providing cleaner data quicker and providing up-to-date interim progress reports in a timely manner.

Listed below are some of the steps involved in integrating the communication component before to, during, and after data collection as well as data management.

Electronic Based Systems:

Electronic-based data collection and management systems have brought about a significant transformation in the field of data collection and management. These systems offer substantial advantages over traditional paper-based methods, particularly in terms of efficiency and accessibility. The advantages encompass quick access to real-time data, enabling timely decision-making for relevant stakeholders. Additionally, these systems facilitate easy monitoring of protocol adherence, enrolment rates, and performance metrics at various participating sites. The following categories illustrate the diversity within electronic-based systems:

Centralized Systems

Distributed Systems

Wireless Systems

PDF-Based Systems

Web-Based Systems

Direct Systems

These electronic systems typically incorporate integrated components utilizing diverse technologies, enabling flexible data entry, submission, and management methods. Alternatively, CROs may choose from a variety of industry suppliers that provide well-established proprietary data gathering and administration systems, often known as e-clinical software. Instead of building systems in-house, this gives you an option. Oracle Clinical v4i®, DataLabsXC®, TrialMaster®, and ClinPlus® Data Management (CPDM) are some well-known examples of e-clinical software. These applications were created by several companies. The many features offered by these software systems address the unique requirements of clinical research data administration and collecting.

Processes before Data Collection:

Proper development of procedure, determining the type of data to be collected, defining procedures for subject recruitment, registration, screening, randomization, and treatment dispensing are the first steps in data collection. In a broader sense data collection in loves two steps i.e. 1) Choosing a Data Collection and Management System 2) Hardware and Software Selection.

Processes during Data Collection:

1. **Ensuring Data Quality**: Ensuring the trial's integrity and effective conclusion requires constant monitoring during data gathering. This work has been made easier with the development of

specialized computer software and applications. Trial staff are able to react efficiently to any development thanks to these technologies. Creating individualized routines that generate monitoring reports is an important part of clinical trial monitoring.

2. **Treatment Dispensing**: The distribution of medications or equipment to facilities participating in clinical trials requires a reliable system. It is critical to use individuals' randomization numbers to assign the right medication regimens or devices. In this procedure, computers are crucial for ensuring that distribution is done accurately and on schedule. Accurate record-keeping of dispensed and returned products is made possible by the computer systems used by the pharmacy coordinating center, which monitor the distribution status at each location.
3. **Handling Unexpected Events**: Unexpected events may arise during the course of a clinical trial, necessitating swift action. Some situations may require adjustments to the data collection and management system. For instance, if a subject relocates to another participating site but wishes to continue participation, their records must be transferred from the previous site. The approach to accomplish this depends on the type of data collection and management system in place.
4. **Data Transformation**: In order to improve the efficiency and precision of reporting trial results, several computer applications and programs have been created to simplify the process of transforming, manipulating, and analyzing trial data. Data transformation is essential when the extracted data cannot be used directly in the analysis program. To transform acquired data from its initial format into the one needed for analysis, there are a plethora of data conversion software programs to choose from. This guarantees that the analysis phase will be seamlessly integrated.

Process after Data Collection

1. **Data Lockdown**: Despite its importance and the need for careful preparation for a prompt and orderly conclusion, the practicalities of shutting down big, multicenter clinical trials have gotten little attention.
2. **Data Retention**: For the sake of future reference, it is essential that all data gathered at each location be saved securely in a read-only manner. After the study ends, each site's Institutional Review Board (IRB) must preserve the local database.

3. **Data Archiving**: After a clinical trial's data collection and analysis are complete, the coordinating institution usually archives all of the obtained data for future reference. The data gathering system used determines the technique of data archiving. Paper forms may need to be preserved for a certain amount of time when data is collected using paper-based methods..

4. **Facilitating Data Sharing**: Computers play a pivotal role in facilitating data sharing among researchers. Leveraging the Internet, data repositories for completed clinical trials can be effectively designed and implemented. Repository software can categorize users, granting administrative users full access to the repository.

   The United States Federal Regulation known as 21 CFR Part 11 concentrates on electronic records. The evolution from primitive, uncontrolled manufacturing processes led the FDA to establish "Good Manufacturing Practices," subsequently followed by "Good Laboratory Practices," "Good Clinical Practices," and "Good Tissue Practices." Together, these practices set industry standards. Biopharmaceutical companies are "self-regulated," according to the FDA, which means they are responsible for their own regulation but still has the power to guarantee and monitor compliance.

Regulations of Computer Systems

It is the duty of the regulated entity to determine whether a system does not fit within the high-risk requirement circle and to provide justification for this determination. Part 11 is now mandatory for high-risk systems that have an impact on human health and safety and acts as a guideline for industrial management of all computer systems. The legislation combined criteria for system validation and all prior advice relating to computer systems. It also offered direction for electronic record preservation and electronic signature approval, with an emphasis on the approval and long-term inspection of such records.

Bibliography

1. Approaches for the Application of Physiologically-Based Pharmacokinetic (PBPK)Models and Supporting Data in Risk Assessment E-Docket ID No.ORD-2005-0022. *Fed Reg* July 28, 2005; 70 (144): 43692–43693 .
2. Computer simulation in pharmacokinetic and pharmacodynamic studies. *Durgawati Patel and Puspendra Kumar,* September 22, 2017.

3. Computer simulations in pharmacokinetics and pharmacodynamics: Rediscovering systems physiology in the 21st century. *Paolo vicini,2006;21:513-527.*
4. Gieschke R, Reigner BG, Steimer JL. Exploring clinical study design by computer Simulation based on pharmacokinetic/ pharmacodynamic modelling.*Int J Clin Pharmacol Ther* 1997;35: 469–74.
5. Sheiner LB, Ludden TM. Population pharmacokinetics/ dynamics. *Annu Rev Pharmacol Toxicol 1992; 32: 185–209.*

UNIT V

Artificial Intelligence

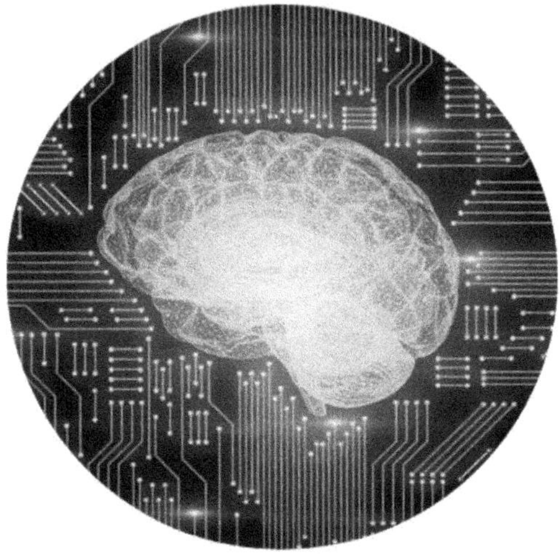

Artificial intelligence (AI) is a branch of computer science that deals with problem-solving by the aid of symbolic programming. A large number of researches are being carried out to improve the current available AI technology to make the pharmacy profession more efficient.

Basic component of AI

1. Deep learning
2. Machine learning
3. Computer vision
4. Cognitive computing
5. Natural learning processing
6. Neural network

AI has a long history, dating back to its proposal at the Dartmouth Conference in 1956. It was described at the time as an algorithm that gives robots the capacity to think for themselves and carry out numerous tasks. Support vector machines (SVM) and artificial neural networks (ANN) are two examples of the cutting edge technology that have emerged as a result of AI's development from its perceptual machine roots. Despite facing some challenges and setbacks, AI has seen significant progress, particularly due to the availability of advanced hardware support.

In the realm of computer science, AI is considered a branch that focuses on problem-solving using symbolic programming. It has the potential to revolutionize various industries, including pharmacy. A considerable amount of research is being conducted to enhance the current AI technology, aiming to make the pharmacy profession more efficient and effective by discovering the new drug molecule along with its formulation and optimization parameters. The integration of AI in pharmaceutical research and development can lead to significant advancements and streamlined processes, ultimately benefiting patient care and the healthcare industry as a whole [1]. In a broader senses the main components of AI are Deep learning, Machine learning, Computer vision, Cognitive computing and Artificial neural network (ANN).

Machine learning has a branch called deep learning. The human brain's biological neural networks serve as inspiration for these artificial neural networks, which are designed to function similarly to the way those neurons in the brain process data. They are capable of determining a single output from multiple inputs by using multiple layers of networks that work together. Positive and negative reinforcement are used in the learning process of deep learning, which needs continuous processing and reinforcement to make progress. One area where deep learning has been put to use is in automatic voice identification and translation. It can also be applied in manufacturing processes, such as drug formulation and monitoring, to streamline operations and reduce human intervention.

Machine learning, on the other hand, is a more general use of AI that relies on specially programmed computers to do a variety of tasks. Without the need for manual coding, it enables systems to automatically learn and improve as they go along. Healthcare, pharmacology, and the biological sciences are just a few of the many fields that might benefit from machine learning. In the pharmaceutical industry, machine learning is used for tasks such as grinding, mixing, granulating, drying, filling, packing, and testing. It is also widely used in analytical testing, such as HPLC, HPTLC, NMR, DSC, and TGA. Moreover, machine learning is employed in genetic data sequencing, coding, and data recognition to develop biomedicines. Graphs, tables, photographs, and other text and video may all be understood with the help of computer vision, a branch of AI that use deep learning and pattern recognition to decipher the information contained inside PDF documents which is utilised to speed up patient diagnoses by analysing x-rays. Computer vision is also applied to identify chemical components, formulate complexation, and analyze genetic structures.

Cognitive computing is another aspect that aims to recreate the human thought process in a computer model. The goal of cognitive computing is to simulate human reasoning in a digital environment. Human language and the interpretation of visuals are essential to this. Coupling human-like behaviour with advanced computational and information processing capabilities, this is the goal of cognitive computing and artificial intelligence. Teaching robots to comprehend human language in context and respond sensibly is meant to pave the way for frictionless interactions between people and technology.

Artificial neural network (ANN) model involves computations and mathematics, which simulate the human–brain processes as shown in figure 1. By combining experimental and evidence-based data during drug discovery, ANN is able to tackle complex difficulties in the drug discovery process by absorbing information and drawing meaningful conclusions from Quantitative structure-activity relationship (QSAR), quantitative structure-toxicity relationship (QSTR), pharmacokinetics, and pharmacodynamic studies, docking, formulation development, design of chemical synthesis, and high-throughput screening (HTS) study.

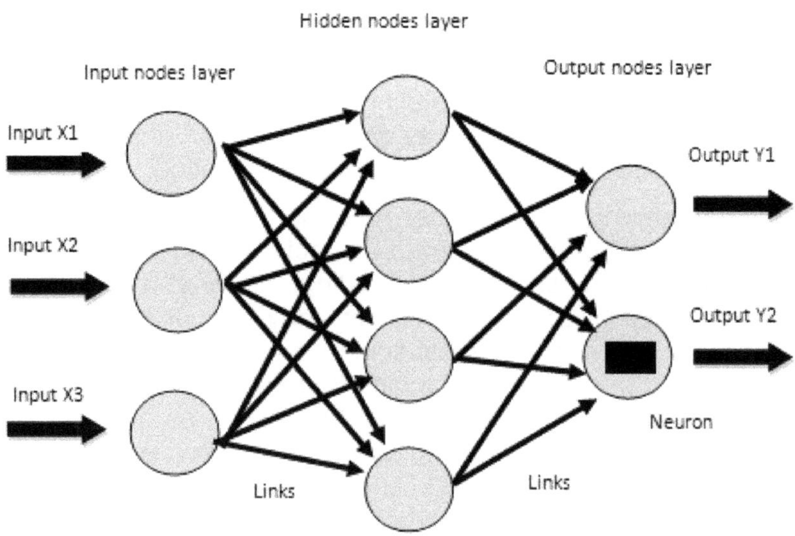

FIGURE 1 Basic of artificial neural network.

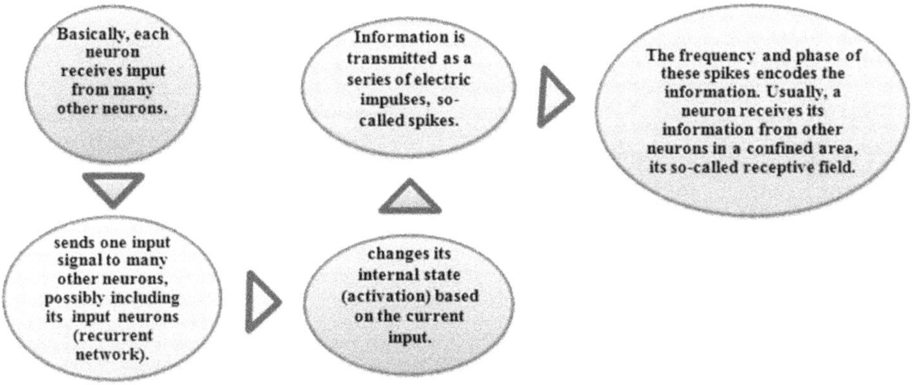

FIGURE 2 Working step of artificial neural network.

Integration of AI in Manufacturing Execution Systems (MES)

Manufacturing Execution Systems (MES) serve as control systems meticulously designed to real-time manage, monitor, and track diverse manufacturing information. Data is continuously gathered from sources like robots, employees, and machine monitors. Currently, MES is extensively fused with enterprise resource planning systems, allowing seamless integration. MES ensures adherence to regulatory guidelines while maintaining the production of high-quality products. The utilization of MES offers several advantages, including guaranteed legal compliance, risk reduction, enhanced transparency, streamlined production cycles, optimal resource allocation, monitored production stages, and optimization leading up to batch release [2-5].

Incorporating AI in Automated Control Process Systems (ACPS)

Automated Control Process Systems (ACPS) play a pivotal role in ensuring the safe and profitable execution of processes. Constant monitoring of process variables such as temperature, pressure, flow, vacuum, and concentration is conducted. When necessary, prompt actions such as adjusting pump speeds, valve openings, or heater settings are taken to maintain required variables. ACPS offers notable advantages, including achieving superior quality at reduced costs, material savings, ensuring personnel and plant safety, boosting yield, and lowering labor expenses.

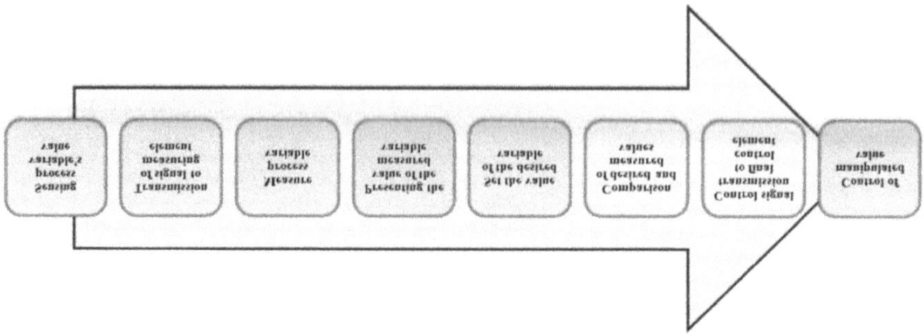

FIGURE 3 Process of ACPS.

Importance of AI in Pharmacy

1. **Enhanced Data Analysis and Pharmacological Research**

   AI exhibits the capacity to identify nonlinear relationships within noisy datasets. Spectral data analysis of multi component samples is streamlined, facilitating the detection and calibration of structurally similar amino acids like tyrosine and tryptophan. Moreover, AI aids in determining the concentration of chiral compounds and enantiomers. The application of diffuse reflectance IR spectral data and X-ray diffraction assists in sensitive identification of ranitidine-HCL. Optimal gradient conditions for anion separation in chromatography are efficiently selected.

2. **Advancements in Preformulation**

   AI contributes to comprehending the physicochemical processes of amorphous polymers. Predictions of water uptake, glass transition temperature, and viscosity are made with minimal prediction errors. The relationship between polymer blend composition and water uptake profiles, as well as viscosity of polymer solutions, is effectively established. Moisture content's influence on polymer glass transition temperature is identified. AI facilitates the assessment of API impact on tablet properties and designing stable formulations for multiple active components, thus reducing preformulation study duration and costs.

3. **Optimization of Pharmaceutical Formulations**

   AI's predictive capabilities are harnessed through polynomial equations and response surface methodologies for pharmaceutical response prediction and optimization. Pharmacokinetic simulation aids in controlled release formulation design. The effects of variables such as coating weight gain, curing duration, and plasticizer concentration on in-vitro drug release data are assessed. Process and formulation variables like drug amount, osmotic pressure of promoting agents, polymer content, and coating weight are also investigated.

4. ***In Vitro-In Vivo* Correlation (IVIVC)**

   IVIVC assists in predicting salbutamol absorption in healthy and asthmatic volunteers' lungs through urine drug concentration and lung function comparison. Hepatocyte-based in-vitro data helps for

5. **Quantitative Structural Relationship and Property Relationship**

   AI effectively correlates compound descriptors with chemical, biological activities, and physicochemical properties based on molecular structures. QSAR studies rely on the independence of biological activities from physicochemical parameters. Pharmacokinetic parameters are predicted using octanol-water partition coefficients and pKa functions bound to plasma proteins. The relationship between tissue distribution lipophilicity of homogenous compounds is calculated using a mechanistic model and an empirical ANN model, aiding in ADMET prediction.

6. **In Proteomics and Genomics**

   AI excels in recognizing patterns, protein domains, enzyme class predictions, DNA/RNA sequence classifications, and peptides. The separation of peptides through strong anion exchange chromategraphy predicts peptide separation and protein identification. Folding and secondary structure of RNA strands are determined, and ANN-based algorithms identify, characterize, and predict stabilization centers. Active site recognition and accurate prediction of enzyme classes are achieved for novel protein structures.

7. **Pharmacokinetics**

   AI monitors multiple pK interactions in biological systems and predicts pharmacodynamic parameters like clearance rate, protein-bound fraction, and volume of distribution. Physicochemical properties including protein binding, partition coefficients, dissociation constants, clearance, and volume of distribution are estimated.

8. **Permeability Prediction for Skin and Blood-Brain Barrier**

   AI contributes to the study of toxic compound absorption into animal skin. ANN models utilizing genetic algorithms predict maximum steady-state flux, taking into account molecule size, shape, intermolecular interactions, hydrogen bonding capacity, and configuration stability. Skin permeability predictions are based on molecular descriptors such as molecular weight and partial changes. Blood-brain distribution patterns are recognized and predicted through logarithmic functions, facilitating the construction of predictive log BB-QSAR models based on MLR and SVM methods.

Advantages of AI

1. This is an alternative to classical modeling (Response surface modeling) when applied to variable data set presenting nonlinear relationship.
2. When the neural network fails, it can continue work without any problem by their parallel programming nature.
3. It can be implemented in any application related to pharmacy.
4. It does not need to be programmed.
5. It involves human-like thinking.
6. Also not required rigidity structure experimental design and can be map function using historical or incomplete data.
7. It has the potential for high fault tolerance.
8. It also works on pharmaceutical research including pharmaco-kinetic, pharmacodynamic modelling optimization of dosage and drug delivery system.
9. It provides a general solution with good predictive accuracy.
10. Neural network has an important role in image analysis and signal processing.

Disadvantages

1. **Hardware dependence:** With the parallel processing power, it requires processor.
2. **Determination of proper network structure:** There is no precise rule for determination of the structure of ANN; the network formation is achieved by practice and trial & error.
3. **Duration of network is unknown:** The network reduces the certain value of error on the sample means, as the training has been done but value does not give the most favourable result.
4. **Difficulty of showing the problem to network:** The problem has to be translated into numerical value before being introduced to ANN. The display value mechanism to be determined here will directly influence the performance of the network.
5. **Unexplained behavior of the network:** When ANN produce probing solution, It does not give a clue as to why and how. This reduces trust in the network.

Pharmaceutical Companies using AI

Artificial intelligence (AI) is rapidly transforming the pharmaceutical industry [6-12]. AI is being used to improve drug discovery, development, and manufacturing. Reverse Engineering & Forward Simulation (REFS) is a piece of machine learning software developed by GNS Healthcare that helps doctors automatically match pharmacological treatments to specific patients. It is able to forecast a patient's reaction to prospective medication treatments by analysing a variety of elements that may impact the outcomes, such as the body's capacity to absorb substances, their distribution in the body, and a person's metabolism. This ability allows it to predict how a patient will react to a medicine. For structure-based drug design and discovery, Atom wise has created Atom Net technology, which uses deep learning neural networks. Convolutional neural networks are used, which are also found in voice and facial recognition technologies as well as in self-driving automobiles. Atom Net can learn chemical binding properties without requiring human tuning or over-parameterization since it displays molecule-protein interaction as 3D pixels with channels for distinct atoms. In the drug discovery process, Atom wise identifies regions for potential small molecules and screens them for molecules that bind to specific targets.

In silico Medicine has launched its Pharm AI project, which employs generative adversarial networks (GAN) and reinforcement learning algorithms. New molecular structures may be created and the causes of illnesses can be traced with the use of these technologies. The organisation also gathers and analyses healthy and disease-affected tissue to discover patterns in the ageing process and illnesses, which helps in medication treatment development and drug scoring for efficacy assessment. New and better therapies are developed and people's access to those treatments is streamlined with the use of AI technologies at Novartis Health. Digital photographs of cells treated with various experimental substances are analysed by the company's machine learning system and then classified. In order to help researchers make better use of insights gained through their work and to forecast which untested compounds could be worth examining in further depth, machine learning algorithms can categorise compounds based on their effects. Verge Genomics uses automated data collection and analysis to combat difficult illnesses including amyotrophic lateral sclerosis (ALS) and Alzheimer's. This firm uses search engine-like methods, like those developed by Google, to identify disease-causing genes and discover medications that work on numerous genes at once. Artificial intelligence software developed by Bayer and Merck & Co to aid in the management of chronic thromboembolic pulmonary hypertension (CTEPH) has been granted Breakthrough Device Designation by the Food and Drug Administration. The software analyzes image findings and a patient's clinical history to assist radiologists in identifying CTEPH patients more efficiently. IBM Watson facilitates clinicians in finding suitable clinical trials for eligible patients quickly and easily. Real-time analysis of both organised and unstructured patient medical information is performed by the software, with the result being a summary of pertinent features that may be used by physicians to narrow down the field of clinical trials for a certain diagnosis.

Apple uses AI to improve healthcare by collecting data from iPhone and Apple Watch products. This data is used to create apps for medical research through an open-source framework called Research Kit. Health Kit enables physicians to get data like heart rate and daily step count from patients' iOS devices, which might ease patient recruitment for clinical trials.

The artificial intelligence drug discovery company Exscientia partnered with Alzheimer's Research UK Oxford Drug Discovery Institute (ARUK-ODDI) in developing drugs for Alzheimer's disease.

Similarly Genesis Therapeutics, a biotech company partnered with Genentech, a member of the Roche Group that uses artificial intelligence for drug discovery and development using machine learning and various *in silico* technique in identifying the drug molecule.

Bayer has entered into three-year collaboration with Exscientia Ltd., a UK-based Artificial Intelligence (AI) driven drug discovery company and to carry out research to identify and optimize novel lead structures for potential drug candidates to treat cardiovascular and oncological diseases.

Robotics

Automation is rapidly gaining prominence in pharmaceutical manufacturing, encompassing automated inspection and packaging processes. The numerous advantages of automation encompass enhanced efficiency, protection of workers from hazardous environments or monotonous tasks, reduction in training requirements, elimination of human errors, improved repeatability and reproducibility, and, particularly in clean rooms, mitigation of the risk of human-induced contamination [13-15].

Robotic systems epitomize a form of automation that features multiple axes of motion and programmability for executing designated functions. These robots come in various types, such as articulated, cartesian (gantry), parallel (delta), and selective compliance assembly robot arm (SCARA). An exemplar application includes "pick and place" operations, frequently executed by SCARA robots. Chris Sumner, the managing director of Fanuc Robotics UK and vice-president of Fanuc Europe Corporation, highlighted the rising usage of delta robots for high-speed tasks, citing Merck's application of a Fanuc delta robot to affix dispenser caps onto allergy medication bottles. Sumner explained that the system accommodates ten bottle variants, and switching between them only entails selecting the appropriate program on the robot controller.

According to a study conducted by the Association for Packaging and Processing Technologies (PMMI), robots are projected to manage 34% of primary pharmaceutical packaging operations in North America by 2018, up from 21% in 2013. This expansion of robotic utilization is noticeable across dispensing, sorting, kit assembly, light machine-tending, and traditional packaging tasks. Jonathan Ferrell, a packaging market manager at ABB Robotics, underlines the straightforward merits of robotics, including heightened speed and accuracy, greater flexibility and reliability compared to rigid automation, and the progressively affordable nature of robotic systems.

Use of Robots in the Pharmaceutical Industry

Robots exhibit remarkable efficiency by completing tasks approximately three to four times faster than humans, functioning 24 hours a day. This capability proves highly advantageous for producing substantial quantities of products within short timeframes. Moreover, robots possess the ability to achieve precision levels smaller than a sheet of paper, surpassing human accuracy significantly. Operating at a speed of 120 cycles per second, the robotic systems accommodate ten different bottle variants, with human employees only needing to select the appropriate program for the robots' operation.

Use of Robots in the Laboratories

In laboratory settings, numerous tests pertain to drug research, discovery, and development, often involving repetitive actions such as manipulating fluids and test tubes. Robots are well-suited for these tasks, offering easy automation and delivering a consistent and accurate performance. Implementing robots in this capacity allows researchers to delegate routine tasks and dedicate more time to valuable activities like genuine drug development. Programming these robots necessitates simple instructions, obviating the need for engineering skills among research laboratory technicians or researchers. The precision attained by robots is exemplified by their capability to position 40,000 dots of DNA onto a single microscopic slide, a level of precision unparalleled by human hands.

Robots for filling, inspection, and packaging

Robotic technology finds application in vial-filling tasks for slower speed operations. According to Walt Langosch, ESS Technologies' director of sales and marketing, robotic vial manipulation involves transferring components between stations both before and after filling and pack-off procedures. ESS Technologies is also proficient in handling plastic and glass prefilled syringes across various stages of the packaging process. Langosch affirms that automating syringe assembly, inspection, and preparation aligns well with robotics' strengths. The sterile environment benefits from reduced contamination risks due to human intervention, while heightened accuracy and efficiency in robots elevate productivity and minimize waste generation. Incorporating automatic inspection within a robotic setup provides the advantage of achieving 100% part inspection. Vision-sensing technology proves useful in pharmaceutical packaging for confirming serialization numbers, a crucial aspect to comply with track-and-trace regulations. Langosch highlights that the synergy of robotic precision, dexterity, evolving optical technology, and serialization software creates an optimal automated solution. Notably, color imaging in vision sensors enhances discrimination between differently colored bottle caps, fostering improved object identification and placement by robots.

Robots for producing personalized medicines

Invetech, a custom automation and contract manufacturing company, collaborated with Argos Therapeutics which is a biopharmaceutical firm to develop automated manufacturing systems based on Argos' Arcelis technology platform for personalized immunotherapies. As elucidated by Richard Grant, Invetech's director of cell therapy, the Arcelis platform employs two five-axis robotic arms to produce mRNA from a patient's tumor. This mRNA is then loaded into dendritic cells created using cellular processing equipment. Automation ensures controlled development and maturation of white blood cells into dendritic cells, expressing the desired antigens capable of triggering the immune system to generate killer T-cells targeting metastatic tumors. Utilizing closed disposables, RNA robots execute the process within a common Class 100,000 cleanroom environment, explains Grant. This approach permits the processing of materials from multiple patients within the same manufacturing area, contributing to a significant reduction in facility capital and operating costs. Argos' primary candidate is currently in Phase III clinical trials, and the modular and scalable nature of the automated technology paves the way for commercial expansion. Grant underscores the advantages of robotic scaling, enabling the replication of new sites worldwide with minimal training and minimal variability in production processes between sites.

Clean room robots

Robotic technology proves highly suitable in aseptic filling in industry, as it effectively eliminates the risk of human contamination. The implementation of robotics can establish an ISO 5 environment, thereby mitigating the potential for microbial ingress, according to Langosch's insights. ESS Technologies collaborates with Fanuc Robotics to handle secondary packaging and palletizing tasks in the pharmaceutical industry. Fanuc boasts multiple robots designed to operate within an ISO 5 environment, including the Fanuc M-430iA/2PV. This particular model withstands hydrogen peroxide vapor sterilization and possesses a waterproof rating. Furthermore, its wiring and cabling are channeled through the robot's hollow arm.

Robots created for deployment in cleanrooms must be engineered to reduce the generation of particulates, maintaining cleanroom classifications, typically ISO Class 5 or 6. Additionally, these robots must be designed for easy cleanability, with minimal crevices and resistance to cleaning and sterilizing agents, a crucial requirement highlighted by Grant. Ensuring operator safety is imperative, often achieved through effective guarding or containment of the robot. Moreover, controlling the speed of robot movement is essential to minimize the impact on airflow and particle generation. Additionally, managing heat generation and its influence on the heating, ventilation, and air-conditioning system within the cleanroom is a lesser but still important consideration, as explained by Grant.

Computational Fluid Dynamics

Computational fluid dynamics (CFD) is a powerful tool that can be used to analyze and troubleshoot various process equipment used in the pharmaceutical industry. CFD can be used to predict fluid flow, heat transfer, mass transfer, and chemical reactions. This information can be used to optimize the design and operation of process equipment, leading to improved efficiency and performance [16-20].

Computational fluid dynamics (CFD) is a computer-based tool that can be used to simulate the flow of fluids. CFD can be used to model a variety of fluid flows, including those found in the pharmaceutical industry. For example, CFD can be used to model the flow of fluids in a mixing tank, a dryer, or a spray dryer. CFD can also be used to model the flow of fluids around a pharmaceutical product, such as a tablet or a capsule.

CFD can be a valuable tool for the pharmaceutical industry in a number of ways. For example, CFD can be used to:

1. **Optimize the design of process equipment:** CFD can be used to predict the flow of fluids in process equipment, such as a mixing tank or a dryer. This information can be used to optimize the design of the equipment to improve efficiency and performance.
2. **Troubleshoot process problems:** If a process is not performing as expected, CFD can be used to identify the source of the problem. For example, CFD can be used to identify areas of turbulence or high shear stress that may be causing product degradation.
3. **Develop new products:** CFD can be used to design new pharmaceutical products that are more effective and efficient. For example, CFD can be used to design new tablets that have a more uniform release profile or new capsules that are more resistant to degradation.

Overall, CFD is a powerful tool that can be used to improve the efficiency and performance of pharmaceutical processes. It can also be used to develop new and improved pharmaceutical products.

Advantages of CFD

It has following advantages

1. Investigation of flows that are not easy to measure like Liquid Metal.
2. Pre-calculations for prototypes.
3. Used to calculate dangerous flows (chemical reactions, explosions, etc.)
4. To identify variation in flow parameters.
5. To create a fast and easy change of the geometry.
6. Detailed insight into flow behavior.
7. If you do not have an experimental setup, then CFD is the only choice.
8. An option to validate experimental results.
9. Simulation can be excluded in a shorter period of time.

10. Relatively low cost.
11. Ability to simulate real condition.
12. Provide comprehensive information.

Principle of CFD

It include totally 3 fundamental

1. Fluid static -study of the fluid at rest.
2. Fluid kinematics -study of fluid in motion.
3. Fluid dynamic -study of effect of force on fluid motion

Application

1. **For mixing process**

   A wide variety of mixing equipment such as static mixers, stirred tanks, homogenizers, and emulsifiers are used. CFD methods can be useful to scrutinize the performance of static mixers and to predict the degree of mixing achieved, accordingly indicating whether more mixing elements are required or not. CFD solution can be used to derive the pressure drop, hence the power required. It analyzes the flow field and vessel flow characteristics as well as to describe the influence of impeller location on the flow field and analyze and optimize stirred tank performance.

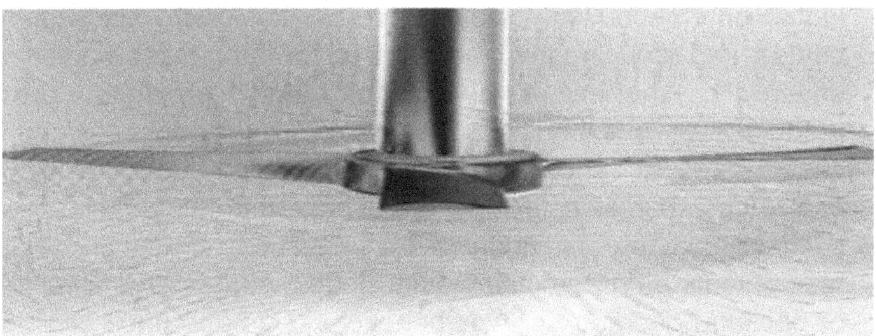

FIGURE 4 Mixing process presented CFD.

2. **For solid handling**

   CFD techniques can be useful to analyze such flows and minimize or eliminate the risk of erosion. CFD also can be applied to simulate the gas-solid flows in complex reactors and analyze the unsteady and chaotic flow behaviour in fluidized beds.

3. **For dryer**

Computational fluid dynamics (CFD) can be used to analyze the performance of spray dryers used in the pharmaceutical industry. CFD can be used to predict the flow of fluids in a spray dryer, the drying process, and the formation of particles. This information can be used to optimize the design and operation of spray dryers, leading to improved efficiency and performance.

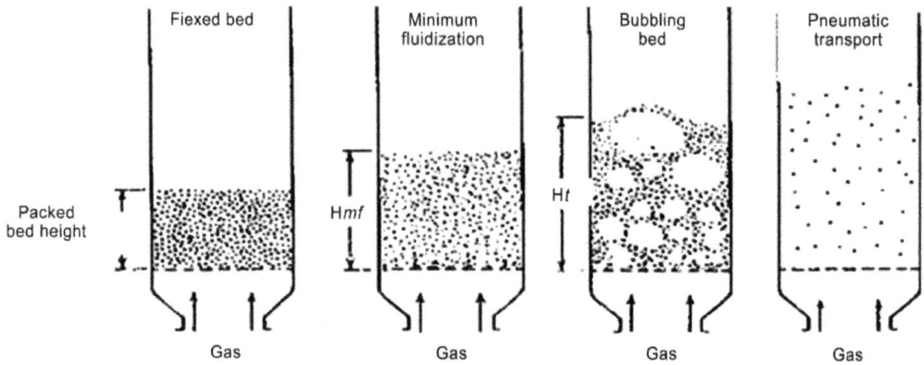

FIGURE 5 FBD presented by CFD.

4. **For packaging**

Liquid pharmaceutical products are predominantly packaged in bottles, and reducing the time required for filling these bottles can effectively shorten time-to-market and enhance overall productivity. To expedite the process, filling equipment can be customized to accommodate different products. However, challenges such as splashing, spillover, and frothing often arise in such filling lines. To address these issues, conducting virtual experiments before implementing modifications to the filling lines or package geometry proves beneficial. This approach facilitates testing under diverse conditions and ultimately results in an optimized filling process.

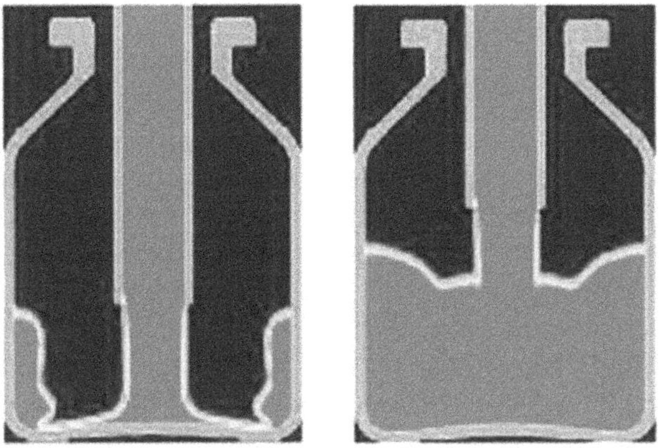

FIGURE 6 Filling operation presented by CFD.

5. **Inhaler development**

   CFD has been used to study the performance of MDIs and nebulizers of various designs. CFD analysis to evaluate the influence of impaction against a grid structure at different flow rates on agglomerate break- up and aerosolization efficiency. Coupling the CFD simulations with in vitro results to predict the actual flow.

6. **Dissolution apparatus hydrodynamics**

   Computational Fluid Dynamics (CFD) proves effective for simulating, analyzing, and gaining insights into the hydrodynamic conditions prevalent in various dissolution apparatus. Through CFD simulations, comprehensive information about hydrodynamics throughout the dissolution vessel can be obtained, in contrast to laser Doppler measurements that offer limited insight into fluid velocity values at specific positions within the vessel. The utilization of CFD offers a unique perspective into the three-dimensional mixing trajectory within the paddle apparatus, a feat that was previously unattainable with velocimetry measurements. CFD is instrumental in exploring the correlation between dissolution rate variability and local hydrodynamics fluctuations. CFD is also employed to simulate fluid flow within the basket dissolution apparatus under different stirring speeds. Additionally, CFD simulations are employed to analyze hydrodynamics within flow-through apparatus (USP apparatus 4), evaluate the impact of hydrodynamics on mass transfer within a low-velocity pulsing flow, and assess the influence of dissolved compounds on local hydrodynamics within flow-through apparatus.

Pharmaceutical Applications

In the Development of Drug Delivery Systems

Increased R&D expenses and decreased efficiency are presenting problems for the pharmaceutical sector in the area of medication development. However, breakthroughs in AI technology and significant increases in computer capacity have the potential to completely revamp the pharmaceutical industry. Artificial intelligence (AI) subset known as "machine learning" (ML) makes use of statistical approaches to learn automatically or via guided instruction. The use of AI tools across the medication delivery process, from initial drug development to stimulating, predicting, programming, and optimising drug distribution in patients, has the potential to greatly enhance the treatment process. Recently, artificial neural networks (ANNs) and other machine learning and deep learning techniques have been used to automate and improve medication development processes and distribution networks. Predicting and manipulating drug release features including solubility, rate, timing, and diffusion at sick locations is possible using ANNs-controlled drug delivery materials or devices. Other uses for ANN software include keeping tabs on drug encapsulation and implanting microchips with medication molecules on them.

Advanced artificial intelligence methods have been implemented to atomize and optimize drug delivery procedures in micro particle based drug delivery. Deep artificial neural networks and Bayesian regularised artificial neural networks have mostly supplanted older approaches like multiple linear regression and multilayer perceptron. The adoption of these newer AI methods has resulted in a faster and more cost-effective drug development process [47]. Similarly in formulation of nano based drug delivery system AI has an important role. The convergence of nanoscience, nanotechnology, and AI is becoming increasingly evident, given the vast amount of data at the big data level. With the help of artificial intelligence (AI) and its subsystems, machine learning (ML) and deep learning (DL), this convergence allows improved data analytics and data mining. AI's processing capability is essential for analysing data sets that include both structured and unstructured components, such as ASCII flat files, CSV, Microsoft Excel spreadsheets, and image processing. Artificial intelligence (AI) plays a crucial part in nanomedicine, which includes cancer cells, biomedicine, and nano biology. Treatment results may be improved, and medication selection and dose determination can be accomplished concurrently thanks to AI/ML and DL platforms. Nanomedicine relies heavily on these features since diverse treatments may be included into nano carriers, and various types of nano carriers can be given to patients with different diseases. As a result, it is clear that the pharmaceutical sector stands to benefit much from the integration of AI, especially in the areas of drug discovery and administration. The convergence of AI with nanoscience and nanotechnology holds immense potential and opens new avenues for the field of nanomedicine.

In Computer Simulation Model for ADME Study

The modern age has been ushered in by technological advancements, and technology-driven discovery has become an integral part of increasing R&D productivity and designing novel chemical entities, such as drug candidates, for use against a wide range of biological targets. Drug candidate failures in the latter phases of drug discovery and development have recently been linked to pharmacokinetic features, often known as ADME (absorption, distribution, metabolism, and excretion). ADME models and AI-driven computer simulations, of differing degrees of sophistication, have been created to solve this problem and aid in the screening of enormous datasets of chemicals. These models have produced tools that are more efficient than conventional methods in terms of speed, simplicity, and cost. Drug pharmacokinetics and pharmacodynamic are studied with the use of computer simulation. A drug's pharmacokinetics (PK) refers to how it moves through your system and how it's used, while its pharmacodynamic (PD) examines how your body responds to the medicine [49-54]. Pharmacokinetics (PK) and pharmacodynamic (PD) are fundamental aspects of drug development and clinical practice in pharmacology. The interaction between these two disciplines plays a crucial role in determining drug efficacy and safety. Over the years, computer simulation has emerged as an essential tool in understanding and optimizing drug behaviour, enabling researchers and clinicians to make informed decisions and design effective treatment regimens. So we may say AI based Computer simulations are used to optimize drug dosing for individual patients, taking into account factors such as age, weight, and renal function. This personalized approach improves drug efficacy and minimizes the risk of adverse effects. Simulation can predict drug concentration-time profiles based on patient data, facilitating therapeutic drug monitoring. By adjusting doses according to the predicted response, clinicians can maintain drug levels within the therapeutic window. Generally there are mainly 4 level of the simulations of pharmacokinetics and pharmaco-dynamic. In Level 1 Computer Simulation of the Whole Organism, two approaches for simulation of whole organism used and these are PK/PD model and PBPK model. The PK/PD model and the PBPK model are two methods for simulating the effects of a drug on a whole organism. The exposure-response connection is modelled using the PK/PD (Pharmacokinetic and Pharmacodynamic) model. A linear model, an E max model, or a Sigmoid E max model may be used to characterise this model, which is paired with a model of a sick state. This model is used to gather *in vitro* physiological and *in vivo* pharmacokinetic data for use in developing a PK/PD research protocol. Pharmacokinetics and pharmacodynamic serve as landmarks on the journey from exposure to reaction. A physiology-based pharmacokinetic (PBPK) model is used to estimate the absorption, distribution, metabolism, and elimination (ADME) of a synthetic or natural chemical substance in a person using a multi-compartmental model that accounts for the effects of blood and lymph flow. Many physiological organs of the body are represented in this model by separate compartments connected by the circulatory blood stream.

Similarly in Level 2 Computer simulations of isolated tissue and organ, Heart, kidney, brain; liver can be a subject of mathematical modelling research which can be carried out with distributed blood tissue model that is known as BTEX model. This is the first ever research on the biodegradation of BTEX (Benzene, Toluene, and Xylene isomer). Benzene, Toluene, and an ortho, meta, or para Xylene derivative make up the new BTEX model. The competitive inhibition, toxicity, and creation of the hazardous intermediate underlie this synergistic and/or antagonistic interaction during biodegradation of the BTEX molecule. The third level is simulation of cell, which is mainly used in biomedical research. Using an online respiratory model, researchers have created a computer simulation of a full cell and made it accessible to their user network. The Cell ML website also provides an online respiratory of the biophysical model. The directed network may be easily implemented on a computer, making it a straightforward method for modelling the intricate interaction between cells or even inside the intracellular milieu. Finally the level 4 include simulation of protein and genes and the goal of this method was to use an ordinary differential equation to map genetic information onto a network, with the hope of identifying the gene(s) responsible for a disease's susceptibility. Clinical data provided significant insight into the underlying disease process, allowing researchers to use simulation to pharmacology in the area of HIV/AIDS treatment creating a novel gene sequence may aid in the protein identification, translation, and transcription.

Current Challenges and Future Directions

Limitations of the Current Methods in Drug Discovery [21-26]

Presently, medicinal chemistry methodologies heavily rely on trial-and-error techniques and large-scale testing methods. These methodologies involve the examination of numerous potential drug compounds to identify those exhibiting desired properties. However, these approaches often suffer from sluggishness, high expenses, and outcomes with diminished precision. Moreover, they face limitations stemming from the availability of suitable test compounds and the challenges in accurately forecasting their behavior within the body. To address these issues, AI-driven algorithms encompassing supervised and unsupervised learning techniques, reinforcement, as well as evolutionary or rule-based methods offer potential solutions. These algorithms are rooted in the analysis of substantial datasets, which can be leveraged in diverse ways. For example, they hold the potential to predict the effectiveness and toxicity of novel drug compounds with enhanced accuracy and efficiency compared to conventional methodologies. Additionally, AI-based algorithms have the capability to uncover fresh targets for drug development, encompassing specific proteins or genetic pathways linked to diseases. This extends the horizons of drug discovery beyond the confines of traditional approaches, ultimately paving the way for innovative and more efficacious medications. Hence, while traditional pharmaceutical research methods have achieved some success historically, their dependence on trial-and-error experimentation and inability to precisely anticipate the behavior of emerging bioactive compounds restrict their efficacy. In contrast, AI-driven strategies possess the potential to enhance the efficiency and precision of drug discovery processes, culminating in the creation of superior medications.

Challenge and restrictions of Using AI in Drug Discovery [27-40]

In spite of the potential advantages AI brings to drug discovery, there exist several challenges and restrictions that necessitate consideration. One pivotal obstacle revolves around the availability of appropriate data. AI-centric approaches typically demand substantial datasets for training, yet the accessible data may often be constrained in quantity, quality, or consistency, thereby impacting result accuracy and reliability. Ethical quandaries also surface as a challenge, as AI applications may raise apprehensions about impartiality and bias (detailed in the following section). In scenarios where Machine Learning (ML) algorithms are trained on prejudiced or non-representative data, the ensuing predictions might become skewed or unjust. Ensuring ethical and equitable utilization of AI for formulating new therapeutic compounds stands as a critical deliberation that requires resolution.

Multiple strategies and approaches are at hand to surmount the challenges encountered by AI in the context of chemical medicine. One strategy entails employing data augmentation, which involves crafting synthetic data to supplement existing datasets. This practice heightens data diversity and quantity accessible for training ML algorithms, subsequently augmenting result accuracy and reliability. Another recourse involves employing explainable AI techniques, which aim to furnish interpretable and lucid explanations for the predictions derived from ML algorithms. This initiative helps mitigate concerns related to bias and equity in AI-driven approaches, while also conferring a clearer comprehension of the underlying mechanics and presumptions governing the predictions.

It is imperative to recognize that existing AI-based methods cannot replace traditional experimental practices and cannot substitute for the adeptness and familiarity of human researchers. AI can solely offer predictions grounded in available data, necessitating human researchers to validate and decipher the outcomes. However, amalgamating AI with established experimental methods can elevate the drug discovery process. By synergizing AI's predictive potential with human researchers' know-how and experience, the drug discovery trajectory can be optimized, ultimately expediting the evolution of novel medications.

Advantages of AI

1. **Reduction in Human Error:** AI can enhance accuracy and precision by making decisions based on collected data and algorithms. It can minimizes errors that can occur due to human factors like fatigue, distraction, or oversight.
2. **Risk Mitigation:** AI robots can handle risky tasks, reducing human exposure to dangerous environments or situations. It minimizes risks associated with tasks such as defusing bombs, exploring hazardous areas, etc.
3. **24x7 Availability:** AI operates without breaks, enabling continuous and uninterrupted work which is more faster and more efficient task execution compared to humans.
4. **Digital Assistance:** AI-powered digital assistants engage with users, offering help and information without requiring human intervention.

5. **Unbiased Decisions:** AI's rational approach eliminates emotional biases, resulting in more objective decision-making which ensures fairness and consistency in judgments.
6. **Faster Decision-making:** Automation and real-time insights provided by AI facilitate quicker and well-informed decision-making.

Disadvantages of AI

1. **High Costs:** Developing and maintaining AI systems require significant resources, including time, money, and advanced hardware and software.
2. **Limited Creativity:** AI lacks the ability to think creatively or generate new ideas outside its programmed parameters. So innovation and unique problem-solving are still human strengths.
3. **Unemployment Concerns:** The rise of AI-powered robots in the workforce could lead to job displacement and increased unemployment and may reduce demand for human workers.
4. **Human Laziness:** Relying heavily on AI for tasks can make individuals dependent and less inclined to use their cognitive skills.
5. **Ethical Challenges:** AI lacks inherent ethical understanding and morality. So concerns about AI misuse or uncontrolled growth leading to unintended consequences like the "AI singularity."
6. **Limited Improvement:** AI performs tasks repeatedly based on pre-programmed data and experiences.

So in conclusion we may say the advantages of AI are evident in its ability to reduce errors, enhance efficiency, and provide accurate insights. However, its disadvantages include high costs, potential job loss, and ethical challenges. Striking a balance between utilizing AI's strengths while addressing its limitations is essential for harnessing its potential in various domains.

Bibliography

1. Arrieta, A.B.; Díaz-Rodríguez, N.; Del Ser, J.; Bennetot, A.; Tabik, S.; Barbado, A.; Garcia, S.; Gil-Lopez, S.; Molina, D.; Benjamins, R.; et al. Explainable Artificial Intelligence (XAI): Concepts, taxonomies, opportunities and challenges toward responsible AI. Inf. Fusion **2020**, 58, 82–115. [CrossRef]
2. Basu, T.; Engel-Wolf, S.; Menzer, O. The ethics of machine learning in medical sciences: Where do we stand today? Indian J. Dermatol. **2020**, 65, 358–364. [CrossRef] [PubMed]

3. Buvailo, A. (2018). How Pharmaceutical And Biotech Companies Go About Applying Artificial Intelligence in R&D. Retrieved from https://www.biopharmatrend.com/post/34-biopharmas-hunt-for-artificial-intelligence-who-does-what/
4. Buvailo, A. (2018). The Why, How And When Of AI In The Pharmaceutical Industry. Retrieved from https://www.forbes.com/sites/forbestechcouncil/2018/04/24/the-why-how-and-when-of-ai-in-the-pharmaceutical-industry/#14bde55c6d07
5. CFD Technology Roadmap, Vision 2020 (US Department of Energy, 1998).
6. Chen, R.; Liu, X.; Jin, S.; Lin, J.; Liu, J. Machine learning for drug-target interaction prediction. Molecules **2018**, 23, 2208. [CrossRef]
7. D.A. Anderson, J.C. Tannehill, and R.H. Pletcher, Computational Fluid Mechanics and Heat Transfer (McGraw-Hill,New York,NY, 1984). PT
8. Faber, K. (2018). How Artificial Intelligence is Transforming Personalized Medicine. Retrieved from http://www. Innovation management.se/2018/06/21/how-artificial-intelligence-is-transforming-personalized-medicine/
9. Faggella, D. (2018). 7 Applications of Machine Learning in Pharma and Medicine. Retrieved from https://www.techemergence.com/machine-learning-in-pharma-medicine/
10. Fanuc Robotics, "A Bright Future for Robotics," Press Release, March 2014.\
11. Gawehn, E.; Hiss, J.A.; Schneider, G. Deep Learning in Drug Discovery. Mol. Inform. **2016**, 35, 3–14. [CrossRef]
12. Gilpin, L.H.; Bau, D.; Yuan, B.Z.; Bajwa, A.; Specter, M.; Kagal, L. Explaining explanations: An overview of interpretability of machine learning. In Proceedings of the 2018 IEEE 5th International Conference on Data Science and Advanced Analytics, DSAA Turin, Itali, 1–3 October 2018; Institute of Electrical and Electronics Engineers Inc.: Piscataway, NJ, USA, 2019; pp. 80–89.
13. Gómez-Bombarelli, R.; Wei, J.N.; Duvenaud, D.; Hernández-Lobato, J.M.; Sánchez-Lengeling, B.; Sheberla, D.; Aguilera-Iparraguirre, J.; Hirzel, T.D.; Adams, R.P.; Aspuru-Guzik, A. Automatic Chemical Design Using a Data-Driven Continuous Representation of Molecules. ACS Central Sci. **2018**, 4, 268–276. [CrossRef]
14. Grebner, C.; Matter, H.; Kofink, D.; Wenzel, J.; Schmidt, F.; Hessler, G. Application of Deep Neural Network Models in Drug

Discovery Programs. ChemMedChem **2021**, 16, 3772–3786. [CrossRef]

15. Grom, T. (2017). Trending 2018: Artificial Intelligence. Retrieved from http://www.pharmavoice.com/article/2017-11-artificial-intelligence/
16. Hansen, K.; Biegler, F.; Ramakrishnan, R.; Pronobis, W.; Von Lilienfeld, O.A.; Müller, K.R.; Tkatchenko, A. Machine learning predictions of molecular properties: Accurate many-body potentials and nonlocality in chemical space. J. Phys. Chem. Lett. **2015**, 6, 2326–2331. [CrossRef]
17. Jarrahi, M.H. Artificial intelligence and the future of work: Human-AI symbiosis in organizational decision making. Bus. Horiz. **2018**, 61, 577–586. [CrossRef]
18. Kassam, A., Kassam, N. (2018). How artificial intelligence can completely revolutionize Canadian health care. Retrieved from https://www.theglobeandmail.com/opinion/article-how-artificial-intelligence-can-completely-revolutionize-canadian/
19. Kleinberg, J. Inherent Trade-Offs in Algorithmic Fairness. In Proceedings of the Abstracts of the 2018 ACM International Conference on Measurement and Modeling of Computer Systems, Irvine, CA, USA, 18–22 June 2018; Association for Computing Machinery (ACM): New York, NY, USA, 2018; p. 40.
20. Kusam, L.; Mayank, D.; Nishanth, K.N. Data Augmentation Using Generative Adversarial Network. In Proceedings of the 2nd International Conference on Advanced Computing and Software Engineering (ICACSE) 2019, Sultanpur, India, 8 February 2019.[CrossRef]
21. Lysenko, A.; Sharma, A.; Boroevich, K.A.; Tsunoda, T. An integrative machine learning approach for prediction of toxicity-related drug safety. Life Sci. Alliance **2018**, 1, e201800098. [CrossRef]
22. Minh, D.;Wang, H.X.; Li, Y.F.; Nguyen, T.N. Explainable artificial intelligence: A comprehensive review. Artif. Intell. Rev. **2022**, 55, 3503–3568. [CrossRef]
23. Novatio. (2018). 10 common applications of artificial intelligence in healthcare. Retrieved from https://novatiosolutions.com/10-common-applications-artificial-intelligence-healthcare/
24. Pearl, R. (2018). Artificial Intelligence In Healthcare: Separating Reality From Hype. Retrieved from https://www.forbes.com/sites/robertpearl/2018/03/13/artificial-intelligence-in-healthcare/#5eb249e51d75

25. PMMI Packaging Intelligence Brief, "Trends in Robotics: Market Assessment, April 2014," www.pmmi.org/files/Research/2014RoboticsPIB.pdf, accessed Nov. 11, 2014.
26. PMMI, "PMMI Talks North American Pharmaceutical Trends at interpack," Press Release, May 8, 2014.
27. R.H. Perry and D.Green, Chemical Engineers' Handbook (McGraw-Hill, New York, NY,1984).
28. S.V. Patankar, Numerical Heat Transfer and Fluid Flow (Hemisphere Publishing Corp.,Bristol, PA, 1983).
29. Schraagen, J.M.; van Diggelen, J. A Brief History of the Relationship Between Expertise and Artificial Intelligence. In Expertise at Work; Palgrave Macmillan: Cham, Switzerland, 2021; pp. 149–175.
30. Senaar, K. (2018). AI in Pharma and Biomedicine — Analysis of the Top 5 Global Drug Companies. Retrieved from: https://www.techemergence.com/ai-in-pharma-and-biomedicine/
31. Shimao, H.; Khern-am-nuai, W.; Kannan, K.; Cohen, M.C. Strategic Best Response Fairness in Fair Machine Learning. In Proceedings of the 2022 AAAI/ACM Conference on AI, Ethics, and Society, New York, NY, USA, 7–9 February 2022; Association for Computing Machinery (ACM): New York, NY, USA, 2022; p. 664.
32. Siegismund, D., Tolkachev, V., Heyse, S., Sick, B., Duerr, O., Steigele, S. (2018). Developing Deep Learning Applications for Life Science and Pharma Industry. Drug Res (Stuttg), 68, 305–310.
33. Silvia, H.; Carr, N. When Worlds Collide: Protecting Physical World Interests Against Virtual World Malfeasance. Michigan Technol. Law Rev. **2020**, 26, 279. [CrossRef]
34. STechnology Vision 2020: The US Chemical Industry (American Chemical Society, 1998).
35. Taylor, L.; Nitschke, G. Improving Deep Learning with Generic Data Augmentation. In Proceedings of the 2018 IEEE Symposium Series on Computational Intelligence, SSCI 2018, Piscataway, NJ, USA, 18–21 November 2018; Institute of Electrical and Electronics Engineers Inc.: Piscataway, NJ, USA, 2019; pp. 1542–1547.
36. Tsuji, S.; Hase, T.; Yachie-Kinoshita, A.; Nishino, T.; Ghosh, S.; Kikuchi, M.; Shimokawa, K.; Aburatani, H.; Kitano, H.; Tanaka, H. Artificial intelligence-based computational framework for drug-target prioritization and inference of novel repositionable drugs for Alzheimer's disease. Alzheimer Res. Ther. **2021**, 13, 92. [CrossRef]

37. Vamathevan, J.; Clark, D.; Czodrowski, P.; Dunham, I.; Ferran, E.; Lee, G.; Li, B.; Madabhushi, A.; Shah, P.; Spitzer, M.; et al. Applications of machine learning in drug discovery and development. Nat. Rev. Drug Discov. **2019**, 18, 463–477. [CrossRef]

38. Wess, G.; Urmann, M.; Sickenberger, B. Medicinal Chemistry: Challenges and Opportunities. Angew. Chem. Int. Ed. **2001**, 40, 3341–3350. [CrossRef]

39. WuXi Global Forum Team. (2018). Artificial Intelligence Already Revolutionizing Pharma. Retrieved from http://www.pharmexec.com/artificial-intelligence-already-revolutionizing-pharma

40. Zaidi, D. (2018). The 3 most valuable applications of AI in health care. Retrieved from https://venturebeat.com/2018/04/22/the-3-most-valuable-applications-of-ai-in-health-care/

www.ingramcontent.com/pod-product-compliance
Ingram Content Group UK Ltd.
Pitfield, Milton Keynes, MK11 3LW, UK
UKHW020046200726
13845UKWH00044B/10

9 789348 734228